# Attention, Voluntary Contraction and Event-Related Cerebral Potentials

# Progress in
# Clinical Neurophysiology

Vol. 1

Series Editor: JOHN E. DESMEDT

M.D., Professor of Neurophysiology and of Pathophysiology of the Nervous System, Director of the Brain Research Unit, University of Brussels, Brussels

S. Karger · Basel · München · Paris · London · New York · Sydney

# Attention, Voluntary Contraction and Event-Related Cerebral Potentials

Editor: John E. Desmedt

95 figures and 6 tables, 1977

S. Karger · Basel · München · Paris · London · New York · Sydney

# Progress in Clinical Neurophysiology

Cataloging in Publication
    Attention, voluntary contraction, and event-related cerebral potentials
    Editor: JOHN E. DESMEDT. – Basel, New York: Karger, 1977
    (Progress in clinical neurophysiology; v. 1)
    1. Brain – physiology    2. Attention    3. Movement    4. Electrophysiology
    5. Evoked Potentials
    I. DESMEDT, JOHN E., ed.    II. Title    III. Series
    WL 102 P963 v. 1
    ISBN 3–8055–2438–2

© Copyright 1977 by S. Karger AG, 4011 Basel (Switzerland), Arnold-Böcklin-Strasse 25
Printed in Switzerland by Buchdruckerei National-Zeitung + Basler Nachrichten AG,
Basel (Switzerland)
ISBN 3–8055–2438–2

# Contents

Contents

## Abbreviations

| | | | |
|---|---|---|---|
| AEP | Auditory evoked potential | FFP | Frequency-following potential |
| BP | Bereitschaftspotential | IPSP | Inhibitory post-synaptic potential |
| CNV | Contingent negative variation | MP | Motor potential |
| EEG | Electroencephalogram | RP | Readiness potential |
| EMG | Electromyogram | SEP | Somatosensory evoked potential |
| EOG | Electro-oculogram | SP | Slow potential |
| EP | Evoked potentials | SPS | Slow potential shift |
| EPSP | Excitatory post-synaptic potential | SWS | Slow wave sleep |
| ERP | Event-related potential | VEP | Visual evoked potential |

# Preface

The method of electronic averaging with digital computers is increasingly used to investigate, in intact man, the cerebral potentials that are related to sensory, cognitive and/or motor events (Event-Related Potentials or ERPs). This powerful capability has been found to provide unique potentialities to analyse various cerebral electrogeneses associated with cognitive processing in the human brain. However, it is only in recent years that steady research efforts have identified a number of critical parameters that had been neglected in earlier studies, thereby making it possible to establish meaningful data on the basis of more adequate methodologies and better designed experimental paradigms.

This book is part of a comprehensive project to evaluate the state of the art in this fast-growing area, to resolve a number of current issues, and to delineate in detail the essential contributions of the ERPs approach for human cognitive psychology and for clinical applications to patients with brain disorders. The project has received considerable momentum from the discussion workshops of the Brussels international symposium on cerebral evoked potentials (April 1974) which brought into focus the essential developments in current progress and which determined coherent efforts on the part of the many experts involved.

The publication project differs both in its design and scope from the usual congress proceedings which generally lack perspective and depth, and sometimes include verbatim discussion material which should indeed rather be resolved by further studies and, if relevant, be included in a consistent report in order to avoid excess pollution of the literature by unsupported items. The chapters in this and the following books include fresh experimental data which have been stimulated by, and indeed worked out after, the Brussels conference. The general design has been elaborated also by inviting many additional experts to prepare critical chapters in order to ensure that the various facets of each major issue are thoroughly considered, on the basis of the most recent (sometimes unpublished) data that can be tapped by the different experts concerned.

A first volume assembling 35 chapters on the methodologies and applications of visual evoked potentials (with 15 chapters on clinical uses) has just come out [DESMEDT, J. E. (ed.): Visual evoked potentials in man. New developments. Oxford University Press, Oxford 1977]. The present book includes an important report on 'Publication Criteria' drawn up by a working party chaired by EMANUEL DONCHIN. The report should set new standards for publication in the entire area. Essential contributions reconsidering the neurophysiological mechanisms underlying selective attention and slow potential shifts in the brain are assembled, and they will no doubt prove of lasting value to upgrade the concepts of gating of sensory input and regulation of cognition-related cerebral electrogeneses. The model of selective attention mechanisms proposed by SKINNER and YINGLING represents a breakthrough based on an outstanding and consistent assembly of new physiological data which are placed into far-reaching perspectives. These new concepts will be further elaborated in subsequent books dealing with hemispheric specialization and with cognitive processing in man.

The third section of the present book assembles a series of critical papers presenting data and concepts which help clarify many pending issues in the field of the cerebral event-related potentials involved in motor control in man. The resolution of several pending issues and the new data pointing to new developments should prove particularly useful. These contributions will be further elaborated in a subsequent volume dealing more specifically with the design and organization of long loop motor control in man.

Brussels, January 15, 1977                                            J. E. DESMEDT

# Methodology and Publication Criteria

Attention, Voluntary Contraction and Event-Related Cerebral Potentials.
Prog. clin. Neurophysiol., vol. 1, Ed. J. E. DESMEDT, pp. 1–11 (Karger, Basel 1977)

## Publication Criteria for Studies of Evoked Potentials (EP) in Man

*Report of a Committee*

E. DONCHIN, E. CALLAWAY, R. COOPER, J. E. DESMEDT, W. R. GOFF, S. A. HILLYARD and S. SUTTON

This document attempts to specify minimal acceptance criteria for reports of studies of event-related cortical potentials (ERP) in human subjects. The requirements we state are not to be taken rigidly. Under different circumstances, experimental needs may dictate varying degrees of deviation from these criteria. We feel, however, that such deviations should be explicitly justified.

This proposal was developed by a committee constituted by JOHN DESMEDT with EMANUEL DONCHIN as chairman. The committee exchanged lengthy correspondence, met in Brussels and presented some of the issues for general discussion by the participants of the International Symposium on Cerebral Evoked Potentials in Man held in Brussels in 1974.

### Subjects

The number of subjects used, their sex and age range must be specified. Specify also the degree to which the subject had had previous experience in EP or other laboratory experiments.

#### 1. What is a 'Normal' Subject

The term normal subject is frequently used rather loosely. Even though detailed information about the neurological status need not to be given in print, a number of features should be checked and reported, particularly if they bear upon the specific experiment. For example, it is useful to know in auditory studies the auditory threshold at 1 kHz. The visual acuity (possible amblyopia), visual field, color sensitivity (evidence of color blindness) and eye dominance are relevant in visual evoked potential (VEP) studies [cf. Methodology Report for VEP in DESMEDT, 1977]. For somatosensory studies, the presence or absence of disorders in skin sensation and of any history of bone fractures, trauma, or neuropathy must be evaluated before a subject is described as 'normal'.

Enquiry into a possible history of brain disease or epilepsy may also be useful. For neonates and infants, the neurological status at birth and the Apgar score should be reported. For subjects above 50 years, the incidence of neurological changes associated with aging should be considered.

## 2. Recruitment of Subjects

The mode of recruitment of subjects should be stated. It is important to know if subject belong to the laboratory staff, are the experimenters themselves, volunteer or paid individuals, patients in a hospital, or ambulatory outpatients. The subjects may submit to the experiment for different reasons. The extent of the subjects' motivation to participate and to perform assigned tasks should be explained. Payment given for the session and possible bonuses given for successful performance in psychological tasks should also be included.

## 3. Subject Handedness

In any study in which cross hemispheric comparisons of any sort are to be made, it is useful to specify the subject's handedness. This is also of interest in studies in which motor responses, by the right or the left hand, plays a significant role. Handedness is difficult to measure and sophisticated methods for its determination are required in studies concerned with hemispheric specialization. (Investigators should at least report whether the subjects perceive themselves as right- or left-handed; which hand they use for writing, cutting ..., which foot they use to kick a ball ..., etc.).

## 4. Drugs

Whenever possible, the use of drugs by normal subjects should be ascertained and reported (stimulants, narcotics, neurotropic drugs ...) as well as for patients under medical treatment (for example, epileptics with barbiturates or hydantoines; Parkinson patients with L-dopa; psychiatric patients with psychtropic drugs ...). In certain cases, the EP study may require sedation, e.g. in turbulent children (Seconal suppositories) or in tense patients.

*Physical Environment*

Describe the setting in which the subject was tested: Ambient room light and ambient noise in the laboratory are important, as is the subject's posture during the test. The location of the experimental apparatus relative to the subject should be described.

*Stimuli*

Provide physical specifications of all stimuli used: Stimulus intensity, stimulus duration, the specific manner in which stimuli were generated and presented as well as the manner of stimulus scheduling should be specified. All temporal parameters, such as interstimulus and intertrial intervals, and their distribution, must be clearly specified. With respect to stimulus intensity, it is useful to specify psychometric information in addition to the physical specifications of the stimulus. Thus, somatic stimuli should be specified in milliamperes above absolute or thumb twitch threshold; auditory stimuli should be specified in dB above absolute threshold (sensation level; SL).

The impedance of somatic stimulating electrodes should be measured, monitored, and specified especially when using constant current devices for two reasons: (1) a large impedance requires a large voltage to maintain current flow which may give stimulus artifact problems, and (2) constant current devices have a 'compliance limit', that is an upper limit of electrode impedance beyond which the available voltage becomes insufficient to maintain the constant current.

While it is necessary to state precisely that a visual stimulus subtended a certain number of degrees at the retina at a certain number of millilamberts, it is useful to also indicate the intensity log units above the absolute threshold for the same stimulus presentation equipment.

*Electrodes*

The composition of the electrodes and the manner of their application should be specified. The electrode impedance, and the way in which elctrode resistance was measured should be described. The monitoring of electrode resistance is important to ascertain the extent to which the original resistance was maintained throughout an experiment of long duration.

EP investigators agree increasingly that they should use as many electrodes as they can in any one experiment, because different EP components may have different scalp distributions. The choice of placements must take into account both the specific goals of the experiment and the number of recording channels available. For experiments dealing with the relationship between EPs and complex psychological processes, a ranking of electrode placements in order of desirability is excerpted here: '... the electrode ranking we suggest is that EOG and Cz be always recorded following which P3 and P4 (or Pz), C3 and C4, then F3 and F4 (or Fz) and $O_1$ and $O_2$, or $O_1$ by itself. If the investigator has channels to spare, placements at T5 or T6 can be made though we seriously doubt the usefulness of these placements.'

To foster interlaboratory communication, this committee recommends that the International 10–20 electrode placement system be used to specify placement whenever possible [JASPER, 1958]. Any placements which deviate from the 10–20 system can still be described in relation to the 10-20 system (e.g. one may report a placement '1 cm anterior and 1 cm above $C_4$', rather than as being '5 cm up and 1 cm anterior to the interaural line'). We recognize that on many occasions investigators have good scientific reasons to deviate from the 10-20 system. We feel that the results would be better communicated if also specified in terms of a standard coordinate system.

When recording montages are used in which each electrode is referred to a common reference, there remains the vexing question of the choice of a reference electrode. In the CNV/P300 area, there seems to be a preference for linked-ears rather than linked-mastoid electrodes. In other areas of research the choices vary widely. The committee recommends that whatever the reference site chosen, the authors should not take for granted the indifference of the reference electrode and they should discuss the choice of reference sites.

Interference from muscle potentials (EMG) can be reduced by avoiding electrode placements which directly overlie the cranial musculature and by obtaining appropriate relaxation of these muscles. Muscle artifacts are especially troublesome in apprehensive and uncooperative subjects or when adequate care has not been paid to securing a comfortable position of body and head.

A most troublesome interference is due to movements of the eyes and to eye blinks. There is a potential difference of about 100 mV between the aqueous humor (positive) and the retina. Any movement of the eyeball causes a change in the orientation of the potential field which affects the scalp electrodes (certainly as far as the vertex) in proportion to their distance from the eyes. Voluntary fixation of the open eyes on a stable target reduces this source of interference, but this method is difficult or impossible to implement in some patients or in infants and children.

The possible contamination from eye movements should be a major concern to all EP investigators and the measures taken to deal with this problem should be considered in any published report. The possible contamination of records by eye movements is very critical in studies of 'slow' EP components. In such experiments, it should be mandatory to monitor eye movements either optically or mechanically or electrically with the electro-oculogram (EOG). Of course, the EOG electrodes sometimes record brain potentials (at the supra-orbital electrode) or the electroretinogram (ERG), but such 'contamination' can be readily recognized. The brain potentials in the supra-orbital electrode increase in amplitude when one maps backwards on the scalp.

The committee believes that it is necessary to average the EOG along with the EP in the same trials as a test for the success of the eye-movement suppression strategy of the experimenter.

### Recording Apparatus

#### 1. Amplification and System Bandwidth

Any published report should clearly indicate the specifications of the recording system, including amplifier input impedance and system bandwidth.

The bandpass of a recording system is determined by the high and low frequency cutoffs which are generally defined as those frequencies at which the gain is reduced by 3 dB (or 29.3%) of its maximum (assuming a fairly 'flat' spectrum). Beyond these frequency limits the gain presents a gradual decline which is described by the term roll-off. If the system includes only one passive RC filter network, the attenuation beyond the cutoff frequencies is 6 dB/octave (the amplification drops by 50% when the frequency of the testing signal is changed by a factor of 2. One could easily overlook the possible presence in the equipment used of two or more filters in series, which will determine a sharper roll-off. Such cumulative filter effects can occur, for example, when the bioelectric potentials are submitted to a first filtering process when recorded onto FM magnetic tape and subsequently to a second filtering when played back from tape to averager.

The cutoff frequencies for a 3-dB attenuation are best given in Hz. The frequency is related to the time constant by the formula $TC = (2\pi RC)^{-1}$. Thus, a time constant of 10 sec corresponds to a low frequency cutoff of 0.016 Hz and a time constant of 1 sec to 0.16 Hz.

When discussing system bandwidth, one must not only consider the voltage attenuation of the amplifier itself, but also the analog-digital sampling rate and the input filters of the averager. When using FM magnetic tape storage of the data, the characteristics of the corresponding electronics and the tape speed are also relevant. All these features must be consistent with one another to achieve an adequate system bandwidth. The system bandwidth should be adequate for the particular experiment considered and no overall recommendations can be made. Bandwidth restrictions may be desirable in certain instances in order to emphasize particular features under study; if so, the point should be made clear in published reports.

## 2. Calibration

A calibration signal such as, for example, a step function of 5–10 $\mu$V should be recorded and averaged using the entire system, if possible utilizing the same number of samples (trials) as used in the experiment. This will give an accurate calibration since it will be subjected to the same rounding errors as the EP. The duration of the calibrating square wave should be about 1/4 or 1/2 of the epoch averaged. Such a record when published would allow a reader to evaluate the systems' effects on the signal. Alternatively, one can use sine waves at different frequencies; however, this would not seem an easily instrumented alternative in several areas of EP applications (for example in clinical work).

## 3. Amplitude Measurements

The method used for measuring the peak amplitude of EP components should be specified as is the method for defining the baseline. Ordinarily, a baseline should be defined using a brief epoch preceding the reference event (for example 0.05 of total sweep time).

At the present time, there is no general agreement as to whether the amplitude of EP components should be measured from baseline prior to stimulus onset or as an absolute distance between peaks of adjacent components. Those who measure peak-to-peak amplitudes appear to feel that this frees them from worry over the fact that the baseline, and indeed the whole EP may be 'riding' on a slow wave. However, measuring peak to peak does not take into account the fact that adjacent components may be differently affected by the independent variables; thus, such measures may provide a distorted view of the 'true' relationships.

On the other hand, measurement from baseline introduces special complexities in the interpretation of data, such as when negative going potentials peak at levels more positive than the baseline and positive going potentials peak at levels more negative than the baseline. No general solution can be advanced and when amplitude measurements are of concern, the careful experimenter will not accept a conclusion unless he has examined his data both as measured from baseline prior to stimulus onset and also from peak to peak.

### Digitizing and Averaging

The two critical parameters that must be specified to describe the digitization process are the number of samples per second and the resolution in bits. The different stages of the recording and averaging system must be consistent. For example, there is no point in using an amplifier band-pass extending to 1,000 Hz if the data were digitized at the rate of 250 samples per second.

### Subject's Responses

In EP studies involving motor responses, the response mechanism should be described both topographically and in terms of the dynamics of the response. The amount of force exerted by the subject on the manipulandum should be given.

### The Independent Variables

The definition and measurement of independent variables should be carefully identified and described and circular definitions should be avoided. For example, an experimenter intending to manipulate independent variable X may assume that certain operations have indeed varied the independent variables that he was interested in. If the design is stated in operational terms no harm is done. However, it must be appreciated that changing some physical characteristics of the stimuli or varying the instructions to the subject will not necessarily vary 'attention', 'alertness', 'stress', 'motivation' or 'effort'. It is crucial to demand that an independent measure of the experimental variable be used to reliably establish the degree of control actually achieved over the experimental variables. It would also be useful to debrief subjects following any experiment. The experimenter should try, in as nondirect a way as possible, to determine if the subject's perception of the situation agreed with his own.

## Data Presentation

It is the responsibility of the investigator to decide how the EP data should be analyzed and which aspects of the data should deserve emphasis. The following comments are concerned with the form in which the data should be presented in a published report.

### 1. The Need for Raw Records

All the members of the committee strongly agree that it should be an absolute acceptance criterion for all EP papers submitted for publication that they include actual records of average EPs. No paper should be accepted in which the authors present only measurements of amplitude or some statistical analysis. One can obviously not require that all data be published. The investigator must use judgment in selecting data to be presented in the paper. Figures should honestly reflect the quality of the data collected. On occasion, a superaverage based on all the data from one session may be usefully presented. In any event, this graphic presentation of the data should include in addition to the 'typical' waveforms an indication of the variability in the raw data. Whenever possible, superimposed records representing several replications under the same conditions should be included to give a clear indication of the quality of the recording process.

We do not wish to imply that the display of actual records can substitute for an adequate analysis of the data. The purpose of presenting the raw records is to communicate the nature of the laboratory's recording process. Only by inspecting such records can one get an idea of the care which the investigator may have taken in eliminating artifacts or of the degree to which the EP recorded in a given laboratory are similar or different to those recorded in other laboratories. Furthermore, by presenting a graphic display of the records one can determine with greater clarity the manner in which the investigator identified his components, decided which latencies to measure and which peak-to-peak measures to identify.

### 2. Polarity Convention

It is often suggested that the EP field should standardize its polarity convention. This is an eminently reasonable position. Everybody agrees that it is ridiculous that a large proportions of the published papers present data with the negative polarity up and the remainder present data with the negative polarity down. However, no one has come forth, and no one is likely to come forth, with a rational explanation of the advantages of one system over the other. The usage is sanctified by the experience in any one laboratory and by the ability of investigators to grasp the gestalt qualities of the records when they are presented in the polarity they are used to. In the discussion at the Brussels symposium, the majority of the participants felt that it would be useful to have a uniform polarity convention, but that it is not practical at present to try and enforce such uniformity, as about 1/3 of the participants used the 'positive up' convention. In view of the above it would be required that *in all published figures* the polarity convention would be indicated by a '+' and '−' sign by the calibration signal. Reporting the polarity convention in the text or legends only would be considered inadequate.

### 3. Nomenclature

Another issue discussed by members of this committee has been the issue of the nomenclature of the evoked potential components. In the 1968 NASA Symposium [cf. DONCHIN and LINDSLEY, 1969], several proposals have been made. There has of course been no general resolution and the usage of different nomenclatures for EP components by different investigators is still quite prevalent. There seem to be two major nomenclature principles. There are those who number components by their sequence, such as P1, P2, P3, etc., and those who prefer a nomenclature based on latencies, e.g. P250, N100, etc. The difficulty for either system derives from the fact that variability in EP waveforms from one condition to another often pulls the rug from under the nomenclature. Thus, the P3 label when applied to the 'decision-related' waves may be the third positive component in some circumstances, but often it may turn out to be the first and only positive component in a record. On the other hand, when one chooses to label this component P300 because its modal latency is about 300 msec following the stimulus one is faced with the fact that its actual latency may vary anywhere between 250 and 450 msec, if not more.

In reviewing the problem, it seems that a distinction needs to be made between *observational* nomenclature and *theoretical* nomenclature. We are using component labels in two different ways. We use them when we try to describe the actual data obtained in an experiment. Such nomenclature is used in statements such as 'we have measured the amplitude difference between P300 and P355'. Such statements describe the data collected and their primary function is to serve as a descriptive shorthand. The committee and the conference participants agreed that for this purpose a polarity plus latency specification is more informative than a polarity-ordinal number convention. So for observational nomenclature a polarity plus latency labelling should be preferable.

We do, however, use the nomenclature in an altogether different form when the label is used to identify a theoretical entity. Thus, when one talks of the 'CNV' or the 'P300' component or of the 'vertex potential', one is talking of an entity which one believes characterizes the evoked response and represents some essential physiological, psychological or hypothetical construct whose properties are under study. The conflict between the observational and the theoretical nomenclatures arises from the fact that the theoretical 'P300' may observationally appear as P250, P300, P350, or perhaps P400. One assumes then that all these observational components are realizations of the unique theoretical process referred to as 'the P300'.

It might be proposed that in the future the labelling should clearly identify whether the component referred to is an observational or a theoretical component. Specifically we recommend that whenever one discusses actual components, measured in the actual data, one should use the 'polarity-latency' convention which will refer to the specific latency of a component *for that particular record*. In describing one's data for a group of subjects, in a group of situations, one may use the modal latency or the mean latency to refer to the component. This observational nomenclature will be sublimated by an identifying mark whenever its use is theoretical rather than observational. Thus, $\overline{\text{P300}}$ would refer to the theoretical component which might observationally appear as P350. The following statement could then appear in a paper: 'For reasons X, Y, and Z, we believe that P450 observed in the female subjects is identical with the $\overline{P300}$ discussed in the literature by investigators A, B, and C, and is not the P200 normally terminating a motor potential.' In using theoretical nomenclatures, we should have as free a field as possible. We have fortunately avoided in this area the scramble to name components after people and we propose that we retain this practice.

For certain purposes, it may be useful to follow VAUGHAN's 1969 suggestion that an electrode label be added to the name of the observational components. Thus, a CZ:P200 is a distinct component from a P3:P200, being the positive component recorded 200 msec. respectively at the vertex and the left parietal electrodes. Whether those are equivalent to a P200 is a matter for experimentation. That a 200-msec wave was recorded at the two electrodes is simply a matter of observation.

*References*

DESMEDT, J. E. (ed.): Visual evoked potentials of the human brain: new developments (Oxford University Press, Oxford 1977).

DONCHIN, E. and LINDSLEY, D. B. (eds): Average evoked potentials (US Government Printing Office, Washington 1969).

JASPER, H. H.: The ten twenty electrode system of the International Federation. Electroenceph. clin. Neurophysiol. *1958:* 371–375.

Prof. ENOCH CALLAWAY, Langley Porter Neuropsychiatric Institute, University of San Francisco, 401 Parnassus Avenue, *San Francisco, CA 94143* (USA). Tel. (415) 681 8080.

Dr. RAY COOPER, Burden Neurological Institute, *Bristol BS16 1QT* (England). Tel. (272) 567 444.

Prof. JOHN E. DESMEDT, Brain Research Unit, University of Brussels, 115 boulevard de Waterloo, *B–1000 Brussels* (Belgium). Tel. (02) 538 08 44.

Prof. EMANUEL DONCHIN, Department of Psychology, University of Illinois, *Champaign, IL 61820* (USA). Tel. (217) 333 3384.

Prof. WILLIAM R. GOFF, Neuropsychology Laboratory, Veterans Administration Hospital, *West Haven, CT 06516* (USA). Tel. (203) 933 2561.

Prof. STEVEN A. HILLYARD, Department of Neurosciences, University of San Diego, *La Jolla, CA 92093* (USA). Tel. (714) 452 3636.

Prof. SAMUEL SUTTON, Biometrics Research, 722 West 168th Street, *New York, NY 10032* (USA). Tel. (212) 568 4000.

Attention, Voluntary Contraction and Event-Related Cerebral Potentials.
Prog. clin. Neurophysiol., vol. 1, Ed. J. E. DESMEDT, pp. 12–29 (Karger, Basel 1977)

# Some Observations on the Methodology of Cerebral Evoked Potentials in Man[1]

JOHN E. DESMEDT

Brain Research Unit, University of Brussels, Brussels

Studies of cerebral evoked potential (EP) in man are developing at a fast rate in several directions. Some of the new methods currently being introduced may be more relevant to specific research problems, while others are rapidly incorporated in current uses of EPs. In such an expanding field, it is useful to standardize some methodological features which may have become routine in some groups, but have not been instrumented in others. Techniques obviously cannot be prescribed and nobody should dictate how anyone is to conduct his own study. It is the privilege of each investigator to freely design his experiments and to explore new approaches as he thinks fit to do. Technological improvements and the availability of new equipments or software indeed support vigorous innovation in EP applications. On the other hand, the investigator, especially the one entering the EP area, can be helped in his design if due consideration is paid to a number of factors or parameters which have been found to critically influence the validity and consistency of EP data.

The Committee on Publication Criteria did not specifically take issue with problems of EP methodology, although its final report (see preceding chapter in this book) obviously implies a number of such points since the appropriate precautions or procedures must have been used in order to allow reporting data as suggested in the Report. The present chapter, which no doubt reflects some of the biases of its author, is intended to supplement the Committee's Report by pointing to a few selected items of

[1] The research reported in this paper has been supported by grants from the Fonds de la Recherche Scientifique Médicale and the Fonds National de la Recherche Scientifique of Belgium.

EP methodology which are thought to deserve attention in order to resolve a few of the unnecessary inconsistencies which remain in even recent EP studies, for example as to the system bandpass required in various EP applications.

### System Bandpass

Restrictive filtering of bioelectrical signals can introduce severe distortions in amplitude and time relationships of EP components. The neglect of the limitations introduced by such distortions has led to overinterpretation of inadequate data and to fruitless controversies between investigators using different methodological criteria.

*High pass filtering* is used to reduce baseline potential shifts at frequencies definitely lower than those of the relevant EP components under study. The low frequency cutoff at which the gain is reduced by 3 dB (or 29.3%) below the flat region can be given in Hz. It is also found convenient to express the low frequency cutoff as a time constant TC = $(2\pi RC)^{-1}$ where RC represents the cutoff frequency. TC gives the time taken for a step function input to decay to 37% ($e^{-1}$) of its peak value. Figure 1 illustrates the standard relation to facilitate conversion between

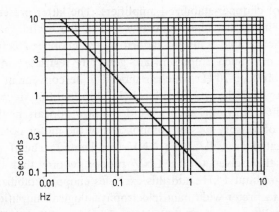

*Fig. 1.* Relation between the two expressions of low frequency cutoff using either the frequency in Hz for attenuation by -3 dB (–30%) below the flat part of the bandpass, or the TC (sec) which corresponds to the time taken for a step function to decay to 37% of its peak value.

these two expressions of the same feature. Needless to say that the system bandpass to be considered must be compatible with the computer sampling rate and filters [DONCHIN *et al.*, this volume].

The choice of an optimum low frequency cutoff in a given EP experiment represents a compromise between several considerations and it will differ in different EP studies. When for example investigating the P300 component or the Bereitschaft (readiness) potential, the system bandpass should extend to 0.05 Hz; that is a time constant of 3 sec (fig. 1). This low cutoff will distort rather little slow EP components with slopes developing over a substantial fraction of 1 sec. A longer time constant or DC conditions might be thought more adequate, but baseline potential shifts will then produce blockings of the amplifier chain which introduces several distortions in the average EP, namely large potential transients at unblocking. Furthermore, if EEG samples corresponding to periods of blockings were mistakenly included in the average, the resulting EP will be underestimated in its voltage. When recording with several scalp electrodes simultaneously, the amplifiers of the different channels can block at different times. Since the EEG samples eliminated from the averages should coincide in time for each of the different EPs of a multichannel topographical study to be meaningfully compared, the exclusion of all the trials with a blocking in any one of the channels may claim an excessive portion of the experiment.

Another way to deal with this problem while actually securing DC recording is by the use of chopper-stabilized amplifiers. The latter present, however, severe problems at the high frequency end of the useful spectrum because the spurious rapid transients added by the chopper mechanism must be filtered out. Such amplifiers are generally restricted to a bandpass from DC to 100 or 70 Hz which is indeed quite convenient to use for CNV studies in which the DC fidelity is helpful to faithfully record very slow potential shifts. However, such a bandpass now appears inadequate if the waveform of sensory EPs or components of the motor potential are to be investigated as well as the CNV (see below). Therefore, studies not confining themselves to the CNV proper require that the bandpass extends up to about 1 kHz and this excludes chopper-stabilized amplifiers. One is led to prefer wide band electrophysiological amplifiers with the bandpass extending, say, from 0.05 Hz to 1 kHz for example for P300 and motor potentials studies. When CNV or very slow potential shifts are of primary interest, the low cutoff can be extended to 10 sec TC or 0.016 Hz (at the cost of some blockings).

*Low pass filtering* is used to reduce high frequency noise. Many EP studies are in fact still not setting a high frequency cutoff by a deliberate choice, but limit this to 40 or 60 Hz by using the readily available amplifiers of an EEG machine. Another bad reason for exceedingly restricting the bandpass is to minimize interference at 50 or 60 Hz from the mains power supplies, which latter should rather be excluded in the first place by appropriate earthing, shielding of the room, common mode rejection and other standard electrophysiological techniques. The current trend at present is to move out of these unreasonable constraints, namely as a result of studies concerned with faster EP components which have been focusing attention on the high frequency spectrum of EPs. One example is the possibility to record and average from the intact human scalp a number of fast auditory component EPs related to the response of brain stem nuclei [JEWETT and WILLISTON, 1971; PICTON *et al.*, 1974; GALAMBOS and HECOX, 1977; MOUSHEGIAN, 1977]. In the somatosensory modality, the neck EP recorded over the cervical spinal cord is another rather fast subcortical component which also requires a bandpass extending to 3 kHz [MATTHEWS *et al.*, 1974].

Such EP studies of subcortical potentials in intact man might have been considered as special applications rather far from practical requirements for event-related potential studies. But this is not quite true since cortical EPs themselves do have significant spectral contents at frequencies definitely exceeding 100 Hz, and which actually extend up to 3 kHz in the case of primary components. This is an important issue in EP research because the 'cleaning' of brain signals by the rejection of high frequencies through filtering not only reduces the voltage of the faster EP components, but distorts them through phase shifts introducing spurious delays in the waveforms. Beyond the high frequency cutoff, the amplifier gain presents a decline called the *roll-off* which is 6 dB/octave in the case of one passive RC filter network (the amplification drops by 50% for each doubling of the frequency of a testing sinusoidal function). When 2 or more RC filters are used in series in the system (sometimes to the surprise of the candid investigator, for example when FM tape-recorded filtered data are played back for averaging, through another system with a filter) the roll-off is much steeper – each RC filter adding another 6 dB/octave. Furthermore, analog reactive filters have come into use which further increase the slope of roll-off and introduce severe phase shifts in the bioelectrical signals [DAWSON and DODDINGTON, 1973]. Neglect for such problems in the literature was noted by the latter authors

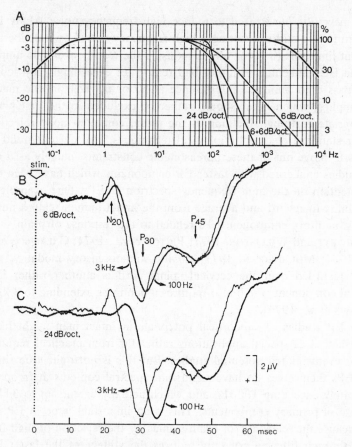

Fig. 2. A System bandpass used, as tested with sinusoidal functions. Abscissa, frequency of testing function. Ordinate, signal attenuation expressed in dB (left) and in percent (right) of the flat response. The dotted horizontal line indicates an attenuation of –3 dB or 30% below maximum. The full line indicates the system bandpass of the system used to record and average SEPs in man. In addition, three different high frequency cutoff conditions are presented, with the addition of filter circuits set at 100 Hz: a simple RC filter circuit (6 dB/oct.), two such RC circuits arranged in series (6 + 6 dB/oct.), and one reactive Butterworth filter circuit of fourth order (24 dB/oct. roll-off). B, C SEPs to electrical stimulation with 18 mA of fingers II and III of the contralateral hand at the time indicated by the hollow arrow. Negativity of the active electrode registers upwards. Averages of 1,024 EEG samples without any ocular blinks or movements or any muscle interference. Nicolet 1074 averager with 80-$\mu$sec bin width and 9 bits accuracy of analog-to-digital conversion. The thin traces were averaged with a bandpass from 0.16 Hz to 3 kHz. The thick traces correspond to the same EEG data averaged with high frequency cutoff reduced by the insertion of either an RC filter attenuating by –3 dB at

who found that in volume 29 of the journal *Electroencephalography and clinical Neurophysiology,* 16 out of the 25 papers dealing with EPs did not even report the bandpass high frequency cutoff while 8 of the remaining 9 papers used an upper limit of only 60 Hz.

In a recent quantitative study, we examined the distortion of early SEP components by different high frequency cutoffs. The main findings are presented here since it is important for the design of EP studies that the frequency spectrum of early *cortical* EP components be truly appreciated. The SEP to electrical stimulation of fingers II and III in 8 normal adult subjects was recorded from the contralateral scalp focus (3 cm posterior to $C_3$) referred to the front (Fz) or earlobe of the same side. Differential electrophysiological amplifiers with 10 m$\Omega$ input impedance and a bandpass flat from 5 kHz to 0.16 Hz (TC 1 sec) were used. The data were stored on a FM Ampex FR1300 tape recorder operated at 15 ips (bandpass DC to 5 kHz). The averaging with a Nicolet 1074 computer operated with 80 $\mu$sec bin width was compatible. For each experiment, the raw data had been edited so as to exclude any EEG samples with eye blinks or muscle interference and 1,024 'clean' sample responses were averaged. The same data were averaged under 14 different bandpass conditions by inserting appropriate home-made filter circuits between the output of the tape recorder and the computer. The high frequency cutoff defined as 3 dB loss (30%) of the peak voltage of sinusoidal signals could be set at 3 or 1 kHz, or at 600, 300, 200, 100 or 50 Hz. For each cutoff chosen, two different filters were tested: a simple passive RC network giving an attenuation of 6 dB/octave, or an active Butterworth filter of fourth order providing a very flat response up to cutoff and a 24-dB/octave roll-off [DESMEDT et al., 1974]. Figure 2A shows the bandpass of the amplifiers without or with the insertion of one or two cascaded RC filters of 100 Hz, as well as with an active filter with 24 dB/octave roll-off of 100 Hz also. The latter filter circuit drastically excludes frequencies above 100 Hz; thus, the voltage of a 300-Hz sine wave signal was reduced to 1% with that filter, whereas it was only diminished to 30% with the RC filter of 100 Hz with 6 dB/octave roll-off (fig. 2A). This is a reminder that roll-off figures are most relevant and should be provided

---

100 Hz (B) or an active Butterworth fourth order filter circuit attenuating by –3 dB at 100 Hz (C). Notice the reduction in size of the early N20 component and the severe phase shift distortion of both N20, P30 and P45 SEP components. From DESMEDT et al. [1974].

along with bandpass in published reports. Figure 2A also shows the marked changes introduced by having two RC filters in series instead of one.

Figures 2B and C present identical SEP data which have been averaged either with the wide bandpass or with a frequency cutoff at 100 Hz with either 6 or 24 dB/octave roll-off (thicker traces). The typical SEP components seen after the thalamic positive field potential [cf. CRACCO, 1972] are the negative N20 (or N1) component, followed by the positive P30 and P45 components [cf. GIBLIN, 1964; DEBECKER and DESMEDT, 1964; DESMEDT, 1971; DESMEDT et al., 1976]. The filters produce severe reductions in amplitude of the N20 component and marked peak delays related to phase shift in all the components, the distortions being most severe with 24 dB/octave roll-off in figure 2C. Quantitative data for the amplitude and the phase shift distortions of N20 are plotted for all the filter conditions and all the data in figure 3. No significant differences were observed between high frequency cutoffs of 3–10 kHz, but definite changes appeared below 3 kHz. The mean voltage of N20 with the 3-kHz filters was $1.3 \pm 0.9$ (SD) $\mu$V. The mean onset latency of N20 for finger stimulation was $18.9 \pm 0.9$ msec, a value which is smaller than that reported in some earlier publications. Please notice that stimulation of the median nerve trunk at the wrist would give a latency about 2 msec shorter than those illustrated here for finger stimulation. In figure 3, the N20 onset latency suffered a spurious increment of 1.5 msec with the 6-dB/octave 50 Hz filter and of 4.5 msec with the 24-dB/octave 50 Hz filter. With the rather severe phase shift and attenuation observed with drastic high frequency filtering, it is obvious that the N20 might very well be altogether missed in EPs obtained under less than optimal recording conditions (for example with inadequate electrode placement, artifacts ...). The mean peak latency of N20 with 3 kHz cutoff was $21.9 \pm 0.7$ msec, and this was prolonged by up to 5 msec with drastic high frequency filtering. The peaks of the positive P30 and P45 components were similarly delayed. The mean peak voltage of P30 (in recordings with the front reference) was $4.4 \pm 2.8 \mu$V [DESMEDT et al., 1974].

The somatosensory cerebral EP with its fast early components readily recorded from the scalp is better suited that the EPs of other modalities for setting a standard about the potentially useful frequency spectrum in EP research. The above data have several implications for current attempts to up-grade EP studies. First, claims about measurements of onset or peak latencies with an accuracy of 1 msec or less can only be meaning-

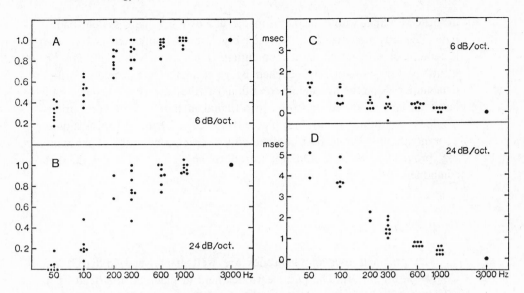

*Fig. 3.* Pooled quantitative data on the relative changes of the voltage of the N20 SEP component (A, B) and of the onset latency of N20 (C, D) through phase distortion for various filter circuits inserted when averaging the same EEG data in the 8 subjects tested. The high frequency cutoff frequencies are indicated in the abscissae. The ordinate scale represents voltage of N20 relative to control (indicated as 1.0) in *A* and *B*, and increase of latency of N20 in msec in *C* and *D*. The values for the wide system bandpass extending to 3 kHz are taken as reference (thicker dots) since no significant difference had been found between cutoffs at 3–10 kHz. Filters circuits were simple RC circuits with 6 dB/octave roll-off in *A* and *C*, and Butterworth active filters of fourth order with 24 dB/octave roll-off in *B* and *D*. Severe distortions are introduced both in voltage and in onset latency of the N20 component by restricting the high frequency fidelity. From DESMEDT *et al.* [1974].

ful on EPs which are not distorted by phase shift and which have been acquired with a system bandpass extending to at least 1 kHz, or better 3 kHz. This point is particularly relevant for studies of EP components which occur during the first 100 msec after the stimulus and when, for example, the latency changes with brain maturation [cf. DESMEDT *et al.*, 1976] or in neurological patients [cf. DESMEDT and NOËL, 1973] are investigated.

Second, in experiments primarily concerned with the slower EP components with peak latencies exceeding about 100 msec, it appears important to be on the safe side in order to avoid or minimize any phase shift distortions which would result from the use of inadequate system band-pass. The true waveform of the relatively fast subcomponents which are becoming of interest in motor potentials, P300 or CNV might not be identified (or subsequently checked by running the same tape-recorded data under different averaging conditions) if the raw EEG samples had not been tape-recorded or stored in a digital memory under appropriate bandpass conditions in the first place. If any high frequency noise should be removed, this would best be done *after* averaging by a digital 'smooth-ing' procedure which would not introduce any phase shifts in the EP components.

### Recording Electrodes

The practical uses of electrodes are well established in EEG [cf. COOPER *et al.*, 1969]. The pad electrodes held in place on the head by a rubber cap or harness are not suitable for EP tests which generally last longer than a standard EEG recording, namely because of the discomfort or pain developing with the steady pressure on the scalp.

*Needle electrodes* are quick and easy to apply and remove. They are well tolerated by the subject in scalp skin and earlobe, especially when they are sharp and thin, and skillfully inserted. The electrodes must be sterilized by autoclaving to exclude the hazard of transmission of viral hepatitis [cf. CONN and NEIL, 1959]. We found it convenient to sterilize sharp stainless steel needles of 8 mm length which had each been soldered to a lightweight female connector (solder junction and connecter var-nished for electrical isolation). The wire leads equipped with the corre-sponding male connector were kept separate and not autoclaved. The scalp skin should be cleaned thoroughly with alcohol before insertion of needles. All needles should be inserted to the same length, about 6 mm, to equalize their impedances. The wire leads should be lightweight and se-cured with adhesive tape at some point on the head to prevent pulling out the needle. Occasionally, it may be advisable to remove a needle and reinsert it nearby, because it elicits local pain or because the pulsation of a nearby arteriole produces electrical artifacts. The hair should be gently parted to avoid contact with the needle metal emerging from the scalp.

Metal needle electrodes exhibit electrode polarization and have a higher impedance to steady current flow than the so-called reversible electrodes. This does not imply that needle electrodes are unsuitable for any slow EP component recording because one must take into account the input impedance of the amplifiers. If an amplifier with 10 or 20 M$\Omega$ input impedance is used, this reduces both the density of current drawn through the metal-liquid junction of the inserted electrode and the amount of electrode polarization. We think that needle electrodes used in conjunction with such amplifiers are quite adequate for studying P300 and motor potentials with a bandpass extending to 3 sec TC (0.05 Hz). When slower EP components are of interest and the amplifier bandpass extends to 10 sec or to DC, then reversible disk type electrodes are required for achieving a consistent recording system. On other hand, if the input impedances of the amplifiers were only about 1 M$\Omega$ (as is the case when using EEG machines), needle electrodes would be unsuitable for recording slow EP components.

Thus, here again, we find a situation requiring a compromise to be made. If a bandpass extending to 3 sec TC is considered adequate, then I prefer high input impedance differential amplifiers connected to needle electrodes which are more convenient to use on the scalp. For TCs of 10 sec or for DC recording, stick-on reversible electrodes should be used.

The *stick-on electrodes* are generally silver-silver chloride cups or disks filled with an electrode jelly, pressed onto the skin and fixed in place with collodion. When of adequate quality, they are non-polarizable and suitable for DC recording. It is generally advisable to clean the scalp thoroughly to remove dead skin and also to scratch the skin in order to minimize skin dipoles and slow electrodermal potentials [cf. PICTON and HILLYARD, 1972]. With the air-tight seal, the electrode paste does not dry out and the electrodes offer comfortable and stable recording conditions. However, the collodion sets hard and is difficult to remove after the session as it sticks to the hair. This can be quite annoying to the subject since small fragments of collodion frequently remain in the hair for some time. The application of these electrodes is also more elaborate and time-consuming than for the needles.

On the other hand, stick-on electrodes are more comfortable than needles on the face and non-hairy skin. They are generally preferred for such areas where they can be applied, not with collodion, but with commercial adhesive disks or with adhesive tape (for example, for recording the EOG or for earthing the subject).

When using either needle or stick-on electrodes, it is advisable to wait about 15 min for allowing electrode potentials to stabilize, thus insuring more steady baseline conditions.

## Eye Movements, Muscle and Other Artifacts

Current progress in EP research frequently leads to focus interest on components or subcomponents of rather small voltage (1 $\mu$V or less) and the possible contamination of averaged waveforms by extra-cerebral potentials then becomes of major concern. For example, movements of the eyeballs rotates the corneo-retinal dipole (retina negative) in the orbits and a downward vertical eye movement generates a negative potential shift at the scalp; this is maximum at the front and decays towards the occiput without becoming negligible though. Such eye movements must be excluded before slow shifts of cerebral origin can be stablished and most papers on slow EP components published before 1972, in which the eye movements had not been monitored, now indeed appear open to question.

The eyes can move and rotate behind closed eyelids. One way to reduce, but not to eliminate, the slow eye movements is to have the subject keep the eyelids open and fixate a point [WASMAN et al., 1970; HILLYARD and GALAMBOS, 1970]. When the eyes are kept open, another problem arises since the subject has difficulties to avoid blinking which produces phasic artifacts. Some subjects are worse than others as far as eye blinks are concerned. Since the potentials' shifts resulting from either vertical eye movements or blinks influence the different scalp electrode sites differently [CORBY and KOPELL, 1972], these artifacts cannot be safely eliminated (as hoped for at one time) by off-line subtraction of a constant fraction of the EOG from the scalp-recorded samples.

The importance of eye movements and blink artifacts in EP studies makes it imperative that the vertical EOG be always recorded and averaged over the same samples as the EPs, and that such vEOG traces be published along with the EPs to permit evaluation of the recording conditions (cf. fig. 4B and C) [cf. DONCHIN et al., 1977].

On the other hand, one might over-optimistically believe that the computer will average out such interferences. The process of averaging only improves the signal-to-noise ratio in proportion to $\sqrt{N}$ (where N is the number of samples taken) provided the background activity is random and of wide frequency spectrum. When the background includes occasional large transient potentials, the situation is by far not so simple. For example, large eye blinks can appear with an amplitude of 50 $\mu$V at electrodes over the central area (fig. 4A). If the EP waveform studied includes components of, say, 2 $\mu$V and if a precision of only 10% is wanted, one should roughly average at least 250 samples in order to increase the

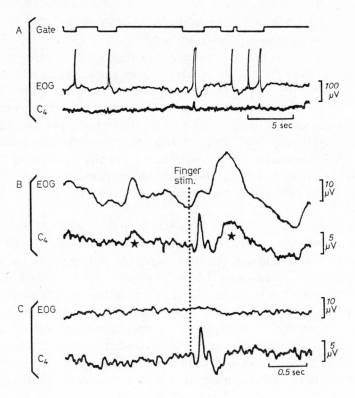

*Fig. 4.* Distortion of EP waveform by eye blinks and the need to eliminate such interference during averaging. Recordings of the vertical electro-oculogram (EOG) by stick-on electrodes placed on the skin above and below the left eye, and of the brain activity from the scalp $C_4$ position referred to the mastoid on the same side. *A* Single sweep at low amplification showing 5 eye blinks which can also be identified at $C_4$ where they present different amplitudes; the upper trace is the output of a gate circuit triggered from the EOG and which is used to select artifact-free EEG samples when subsequently averaging the tape-recorded data. *B* Average traces based on 250 samples showing artifact-loaded waveforms (stars) which roughly coincide with large excursions of the simultaneously averaged EOG. *C* Average traces based on 125 of the same samples after the artifact-distorted data have been automatically excluded by the gate system. The average EOG is now virtually flat which indicates the effective exclusion of the data with eye movements and blinks. The EP recorded from $C_4$ can be considered to represent undistorted waveform. Notice that the amplification is the same for both channels in *B* and *C*. From DE-BECKER and CARMELIET [1974].

relative size of the relevant component $(2\,\mu V \times 250 = 500\,\mu V)$ to 10 times that of *one* superimposed blink artifact.

However, it is quite unlikely that only one blink would occur over as many as 250 trials at the considered latency (with respect to the stimulus or to the reference point in time). The superposition of several large artifact transients will thus severely distort the EP component waveform and increasing the number of EEG samples in the average will not solve the problem if there is any coincidence of artifacts. Practically, one cannot anyway consider increasing the trial number indefinitely, especially in EP experiments involving several parameters to be compared and when adequate intervals between stimuli and avoidance of subject's fatigue must be considered.

The only way to handle the problem is to keep the number of trials at a reasonable level while actually excluding from the averages the EEG samples spoiled with artifacts, spurious transients, and amplifier blockings. Thus, an appropriate channel is to be monitored on a cathode ray oscilloscope and a window circuit with chosen potential levels is made to generate a step function each time these levels are exceeded. One can monitor in this manner, for example, the eye movements and blinks from the EOG, or the electrocardiogram (EKG) recorded by chest electrodes when the EKG is interfering with certain electrode montages (for example, when recording somatosensory EPs over the cervical spinal cord against a distant reference), or the muscle potentials generated under certain electrodes. The latter application is interesting in order to secure undistorted EPs when one wishes to investigate unusual reference electrode sites such as the chin or nose [cf. VAUGHAN, 1969] or extra-cephalic sites; this method provides the experimenter with greater freedom in the design of his experiments since non-routine recording conditions implying more artifactual hazards can be brought under control.

The step function thus generated by artifacts can be used on-line to cancel the transfer of digitized EEG data from a transient memory to the averaging circuits and storage memory of the computer. Even simple averagers like the Nicolet do have provision for using half the memory as such an input buffer while providing circuitry for the conditional transfer to the second half of the memory where the current EP average is stored. Simple circuits can also be used off-line to gate out artifactual EEG samples when averaging tape-recorded data [cf. DEBECKER and CARMELIET, 1974]. These precautions should become routine but, even when they are instrumented, it is still suggested that the vEOG average traces be illustrated in order to indicate in published reports the efficiency of artifact control actually achieved (fig. 4).

### Sensory Stimulation

The brain activity is influenced, not only by the programmed sensory stimuli of the experimental paradigm, but also by all the ambient sensory stimulations not deliberately intended by the investigator. Uncontrolled associations between environmental stimuli and the experimental design can jeopardize the data. The ambient noise should be at a reasonable level and phasic changes thereof must be avoided. The experimental room should thus be isolated from the rest of the laboratory by adequate sound-proofing and it should of course be electrically shielded. Ambient light, if stable, is not critical in most cases. The state of dark adaptation of the subject is of course relevant in visual EP studies. Phasic sounds associated with photic flash stimulation deprives the investigator of the right to claim that he is studying the visual system, since the auditory system is simultaneously activated by the clicking noise of the flash. Appropriate photic stimulation devices allowing the intensity, colour and pattern features to be controlled are now becoming standard, as discussed in a recent Methodology Committee report [ARDEN et al., 1977].

The question of the most appropriate intervals between successive stimuli must be considered in relation to each EP application considered. When the study is concerned with the early components EP (analysis time roughly up to 100 msec), the discrete sensory stimuli can be presented at intervals of 1 or 2 sec. Such relatively high rates are convenient since they allow to accumulate a good many samples in only a few minutes. It is not recommended to use intervals shorter than 1 sec for averaging any cerebral EP, but shorter intervals can be used in studies of brain stem auditory EP, somatosensory cervical cord EP or potentials in peripheral sensory nerves. The above recommendations evidently do not apply to studies specially concerned with recovery functions or frequency-following features of EPs. When the late components of cerebral EPs are investigated, it is recommended to deliver the discrete sensory stimuli at definitely longer intervals, at least 4 sec.

The use of intervals varying in their duration at random in a sequence offers much advantages and should be considered in the first place because it helps minimize cumulative interactions between subcomponents of the successive responses averaged, and it also reduces the incidence of short-term habituation. If one decides to use a given interval between stimuli for an EP experiment, it is definitely better to have random intervals with a mean value of the chosen figure rather than regular intervals so as to avoid these biases, unless there is a specific reason for preferring the regular intervals. Random intervals are readily obtained by using a beta emitter with appropriate circuitry [CARMELIET et al., 1971] or a special circuitry based on electronic noise to generate random intervals with a regular distribution between chosen minimum and maximum interval values.

## Conclusions

This paper considers selected items of EP methodology which appear particularly relevant at the present stage in order to bring more consistency and precision in EP studies. It is emphasized that the report on publication criteria already has obvious implications which are relevant to the use of EP techniques [DONCHIN et al., 1977].

The question of system bandpass required in order to avoid spurious distortions of EP waveforms is discussed in detail. Quantitative studies on the early components of the cerebral somatosensory EPs recorded from the human scalp has indicated that marked reductions in voltage and severe distortions through phase shift are introduced when the system bandpass fails to extend to 1, or better to 3 kHz. It seems obvious that most EP waveform studies should in the future be based on data obtained and processed with a system bandpass extending at the high frequency end much beyond the usual limits set by conventional EEG machine amplifiers. It is also important to specify the roll-off beyond the high cutoff point. The question of low frequency fidelity is also discussed in order to provide suggestions about a sensible compromise between several requirements. It is emphasized that the type of electrodes used, the amplifiers' input impedance, the system bandpass and the resolution of both analog-to-digital conversion and averaging processes should be compatible with one another and meaningful. Different combinations of characteristics have to be considered for the different EP applications, depending namely if either the fast components with high frequency spectrum or the low frequency components respectively are of primary interest in a particular study.

The question of phasic artifactual interferences is also considered, namely in relation to eye movements or blink artifacts which can contaminate the EP components recorded even over the posterior part of the scalp. Limitations of the averaging process are pointed out and it is emphasized that the exclusion of the EEG samples distorted by amplifier overload, phasic potential transients, muscle potentials or EKG by some automatic gating system is definitely necessary if the studies of details of EP waveforms are to be consistently carried out. The surveillance of such artifactual interference by the recording and averaging of the vertical electro-oculogram under conditions identical to those used for the cerebral EPs is necessary to make sure that the EP features described are genuinely reflecting activities of the cerebral tissue underlying the recording scalp electrodes.

It is also pointed out that unwanted sensory stimulations should be carefully avoided by controlling the sensory environment of the subject. Intervals between successive sensory stimuli should be of durations varying at random in the sequence, in order to minimize cumulative interactions between EP components and to reduce the incidence of short-term habituation. Intervals of regular duration in a sequence should only be used when this is specifically required by the experiment considered. The optimum mean duration of intervals depends again on the particular type of EP study and longer mean intervals must be used when dealing with the late EP components of EPs.

## References

ARDEN, G.; BODIS-WOLLNER, I.; HALLIDAY, A. M.; JEFFREYS, A.; KULIKOWSKI, J. J.; SPEKREIJSE, H., and REGAN, D.: Methodology of patterned visual stimulation. Report of a working group; in DESMEDT Visual evoked potentials in man: new developments (Oxford University Press, Oxford 1977).

CARMELIET, J.; DEBECKER, J., and DESMEDT, J. E.: A random interval generator using beta ray emission. Electroenceph. clin. Neurophysiol. 30: 354–356 (1971).

CONN, H. O. and NEIL, R. E.: The prevention of the transmission of viral hepatitis by needle electrodes. Electroenceph. clin. Neurophysiol. 11: 576–577 (1959).

COOPER, R.; OSSELTON, J. W., and SHAW, J. C.: EEG technology; 2nd ed. (Butterworth, London 1969).

CORBY, J. C. and KOPELL, B. S.: Differential contributions of blinks and vertical eye movements as artifacts in EEG recording. Psychophysiology 9: 640–644 (1972).

CRACCO, R. Q.: The initial positive potential of the human scalp-recorded somatosensory evoked response. Electroenceph. clin. Neurophysiol. 32: 623–629 (1972).

DAWSON, W. W. and DODDINGTON, H. W.: Phase distortion of biological signals: extraction of signal from noise without phase error. Electroenceph. clin. Neurophysiol. *34:* 207–211 (1973).

DEBECKER, J. and CARMELIET, J.: Automatic suppression of eye movement and muscle artifacts when averaging tape recorded cerebral evoked potentials. Electroenceph. clin. Neurophysiol. *37:* 513–515 (1974).

DEBECKER, J. et DESMEDT, J. E.: Les potentiels évoqués cérébraux et les potentiels de nerf sensible chez l'homme. Utilisation de l'ordinateur numérique Mnemotron 400-B. Acta neurol. belg. *64:* 1212–1248 (1964).

DESMEDT, J. E.: Somatosensory cerebral evoked potentials in man; in RÉMOND Handbook of EEG and clinical neurophysiology, vol. 9, pp. 55–82 (Elsevier, Amsterdam 1971).

DESMEDT, J. E.; BRUNKO, E., and DEBECKER, J.: Maturation of the somatosensory evoked potentials in normal infants and children, with special reference to the early $N_1$ component. Electroenceph. clin. Neurophysiol. *40:* 43–58 (1976).

DESMEDT, J. E.; BRUNKO, E.; DEBECKER, J., and CARMELIET, J.: The system bandpass required to avoid distortion of early components when averaging somatosensory evoked potentials. Electroenceph. clin. Neurophysiol. *37:* 407–410 (1974).

DESMEDT, J. E. and NOËL, P.: Average cerebral evoked potentials in the evaluation of lesions of the sensory nerves and of the central somatosensory pathway; in DESMEDT New developments in electromyography and clinical neurophysiology, vol. 2, pp. 352–371 (Karger, Basel 1973).

DESMEDT, J. E.; NOËL, P.; DEBECKER, J., and NAMÈCHE, J.: Maturation of afferent conduction velocity as studied by sensory nerve potentials and by cerebral evoked potentials; in DESMEDT New developments in electromyography and clinical neurophysiology, vol. 2, pp. 380–399 (Karger, Basel 1973).

DONCHIN, E.; CALLAWAY, E.; COOPER, R.; DESMEDT, J. E.; GOFF, W. R.; HILLYARD, S. A., and SUTTON, S.: Publication criteria for studies of evoked potentials (EP) in man. Report of a committee; in DESMEDT Attention, voluntary contraction and event-related cerebral potentials. Prog. clin. Neurophysiol., vol. 1, pp. 1–11 (Karger, Basel 1977).

GALAMBOS, R. and HECOX, K.: Clinical applications of the brainstem auditory evoked potentials; in DESMEDT Auditory evoked potentials in man. Psychopharmacology correlates of EPs. Prog. clin. Neurophysiol., vol. 2 (Karger, Basel, in press 1977).

GIBLIN, D. R.: Somatosensory evoked potentials in healthy subjects and in patients with lesions of the nervous system. Ann. N.Y. Acad. Sci. *112:* 93–142 (1964).

HILLYARD, S. A. and GALAMBOS, R.: Eye movement artifact in the CNV. Electroenceph. clin. Neurophysiol. *28:* 173–182 (1970).

JEWETT, D. L. and WILLISTON, J. S.: Auditory-evoked far fields averaged from the scalp of humans. Brain *94:* 681–696 (1971).

MATTHEWS, W. B.; BEAUCHAMP, M., and SMALL, D. G.: Cervical somato-sensory evoked response in man. Nature, Lond. *252:* 230–232 (1974).

MOUSHEGIAN, G.: The frequency following potentials in man; in DESMEDT Auditory evoked potentials in man. Psychopharmacology correlates of EPs. Prog. clin. Neurophysiol., vol. 2 (Karger, Basel, in press 1977).

PICTON, T. W. and HILLYARD, S. A.: Cephalic skin potentials in electroencephalography. Electroenceph. clin. Neurophysiol. *33:* 419–424 (1972).

PICTON, T. W.; HILLYARD, S. A.; KRAUSZ, H. I., and GALAMBOS, R.: Human auditory evoked potentials. I. Evaluation of components. Electroenceph. clin. Neurophysiol. *36:* 179–190 (1974).

VAUGHAN, H. G.: The relationship of brain activity to scalp recordings of event-related potentials; in DONCHIN and LINDSLEY. Average evoked potentials, pp. 45–94 (NASA, Washington 1969).

WASMAN, M.; MOREHEAD, S. D.; LEE, H., and ROWLAND, V.: Interaction of electro-ocular potentials with the contingent negative variation. Psychophysiology *7:* 103–111 (1970).

Prof. JOHN E. DESMEDT, Brain Research Unit, University of Brussels Medical School, 115 boulevard de Waterloo, *B–1000 Brussels* (Belgium). Tel. (02) 538 08 44.

# Reconsideration of the Cerebral Mechanisms Underlying Selective Attention and Slow Potential Shifts

Attention, Voluntary Contraction and Event-Related Cerebral Potentials.
Prog. clin. Neurophysiol., vol. 1, Ed. J. E. DESMEDT, pp. 30–69 (Karger, Basel 1977)

# Central Gating Mechanisms that Regulate Event-Related Potentials and Behavior

*A Neural Model for Attention*

JAMES E. SKINNER and CHARLES D. YINGLING

Neurophysiology Section, Physiology Department, Baylor College of Medicine, Houston, Tex.

At least three separate types of bioelectric events in the cortex of both mammals and man are related to attention-evoking situations: (1) During all types of attentive behavior, i.e. responses to stimuli that are meaningful (reinforced), novel, interesting, etc...., there is a desynchronization of the 8- to 12-Hz rhythmic activity in the electroencephalogram (EEG) in widespread regions of the cortex. (2) During selective perception, the attended stimulus or event produces a cerebral evoked potential (EP) which contains certain components of larger amplitude than those elicited by the same signal when it is not the attended stimulus. (3) During states of expectancy, i.e. following a warning signal that precedes the reinforced stimulus etc...., a negative slow-potential shift occurs, perhaps most prominently in the frontal cortical regions, during the period between the warning signal and the expected stimulus. Thus, when it is obvious to us that a subject is 'focusing his attention' we observe concurrently (a) that he behaves in a definable way that we call attentive behavior, (b) that his EEG desynchronizes, suggesting that the brain is in a different mode of information processing, (c) that some of his sensory EP components are larger for the attended stimulus, suggesting that only certain gates are open for the ascent of peripheral information to the cortex and, finally, (d) that a negative slow potential occurs in the frontal cortex, suggesting that some process is occurring in this particular part of the cerebrum that is especially developed in the human. This paper proposes a neural model showing that these bioelectric activities correlated with attentive behavior are each regulated by two different systems in the cat brain: the mesencephalic reticular formation (MRF) and the mediothalamic-frontocortical system (MTFCS). Furthermore, it will be shown that these two systems converge upon the thalamic reticular nucleus (R), a structure which is a switching mechanism that gates the ascent of thalamic activity to the cortex.

The convergence of the MRF and the MTFCS at R suggests that the three types of bioelectric activity are actually regulated jointly by these systems. Earlier formulations regarding the interactions of the MRF and MTFCS suggested that (1) a balance between excitation of brain activity by the MRF and inhibition by the MTFCS determines the current conscious state of the subject [MAGOUN, 1963] and (2) the MTFCS mediates brief phasic changes in awareness (selective attention), and the MRF underlies tonic shifts in vigilance [JASPER, 1960]. Our present formulation extends the earlier ones and suggests that both systems are integrated into a common system that regulates the thalamocortical activity presumed to underlie the concious states. This paper presents both new data from our laboratory and replications of the previous data necessary to illustrate our neurophysiological model for the gating of thalamic input to the cortex. The next chapter [YINGLING and SKINNER, this volume] illustrates in more detail the relevant events in nucleus reticularis thalami.

## Methods

The new results were obtained in 14 chronic cat preparations with cryoprobes implanted bilaterally in the vicinity of the inferior thalamic peduncle (Horsley-Clarke coordinates: anterior 13.5, lateral 3.0–4.0, horizontal –3.5) and platinized-platinum recording electrodes [SKINNER, 1971a] implanted in widespread regions of the cortex and thalamus. The cortical electrodes were transcortical bipolar and the thalamic ones were monopolar. The reference electrode was implanted in the frontal sinus septal bone. Bipolar stainless steel stimulating electrodes, 0.23 mm in diameter with 0.3 mm insulation removed from the tips, were implanted in both medial and lateral thalamic regions. Each animal had a maximum of 2 subcortical electrodes per hemisphere. All results were replicated in 3–5 of the chronic preparations, except where noted.

Figure 1 illustrates the cryogenic apparatus and probe. Each cryoprobe was constructed of untempered, 0.45 mm diameter, stainless steel tubing with a 0.025-mm diameter silver heater wire wrapped around the shaft so that it could be warmed (DC current from storage battery) to the animal's body temperature, thereby restricting the cooling to the tip of the probe. Thermocouples made of 0.02-mm diameter copper and constantan wire were soldered to the tip of the probe and cemented

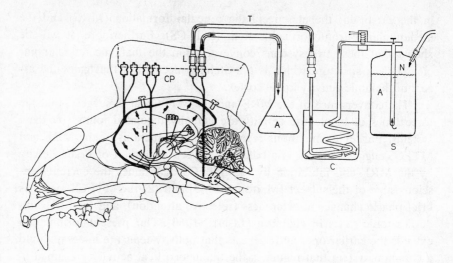

*Fig. 1.* Cryogenic system for producing reversible functional blockade in the brain of a freely moving, chronic animal preparation. A = Ethyl or methyl alcohol (95%) coolant; C = cold bath (dry ice in alcohol) for lowering temperature of coolant; CP = cryoprobe made from untempered, 27-gauge, stainless-steel tubing; H = heater coil, wrapped around shaft of probe to restrict cooling to tip; L = Luer-Lok connectors; N = nitrogen-gas pressure source for circulating coolant; S = steel pressure tank; T = polyethylene tubing to carry coolant to cryoprobe.

to the shaft so as to monitor temperatures of the heated and cooled surfaces. Methyl alcohol, cooled in a dry-ice bath, was circulated through each implanted cryoprobe to produce cooling at its tip. The details have been described [SKINNER, 1970b, 1971a]. All cryogenic blocking temperatures were above freezing to prevent permanent damage and the effects of blockade always returned to normal within 3 min following the cessation of cooling. That the cryogenic blockade is restricted to the vicinity of the tip of the probe has been verified.

The EEG activity and electrocortical evoked potentials were recorded with a Beckman Type R electroencephalograph with 8 channels of chopper-stabilized DC amplifiers, and also on a Precision Instruments FM tape recorder. The outputs of the tape recorder were then averaged with a CAT computer (15 EPs were averaged). The bandpass of the entire system was 0–200 Hz. Monophasic electric stimuli, 0.5-msec duration, were delivered through a stimulus isolation unit by a Grass S-8 stimulator. The stimulation voltage never exceeded 2 V. All electrode and cryoprobe placements were verified by standard histological methods [SKINNER, 1971a].

*Results*

## A. Regulation of Electrocortical Activity by MRF and MTFCS

### 1. Modulation of EEG Rhythmic Activity in the Cortex

*a) Mesencephalic reticular formation.* It is known that brief electric stimuli to the MRF will desynchronize the widespread rhythmic EEG activity of an inattentive or drowsy subject and that electrolytic lesion of this same upper mesencephalic structure will result in large-amplitude 8–12 Hz spindling activity that is localized primarily to the frontal and parietal lobes [MORUZZI and MAGOUN, 1949; LINDSLEY *et al.*, 1950]. However, when large lesions are made in several stages, or when intensive care is given to the cerveau isolé, procedures which enable the animal to survive to a stable chronic condition of blockade, the continuous EEG synchronization is not manifested [DOTY *et al.*, 1959; ADAMETZ, 1959; BATSEL, 1960; CHOW and RANDELL, 1960; SPRAGUE *et al.*, 1961; VILLABLANCA, 1965]. This result suggested that the MRF was not necessary to maintain a tonic state of EEG arousal and behavioral wakefulness, and that an animal could regulate EEG activity without the MRF, as if this system were less important than previously thought. BATINI *et al.* [1959] showed that a midpontine transection of brain stem, just posterior to the MRF, produced an almost constant EEG desynchronization pattern which they attributed to tonic inhibition of MRF by a caudal structure. However, when cryogenic blockade in the MRF was increased in size to include blockade of the midpontine region, the sustained synchronization in the frontal half of the brain became tonically desynchronized (fig. 2B) [SKINNER, 1970a]. Since disinhibition of the already blocked MRF could not have occurred in the latter experiment, brain stem mechanisms for synchronization of the EEG must project independently to the higher cerebrum. Long-term blockade (12 h) of the MRF in chronic cat preparations by small bilateral cooling gradients on either side of the midline (8 °C tip temperature) produced sustained EEG synchronization that reversed to the normal awake desynchronized pattern within 3 min upon cessation of cooling (fig. 2A). Thus, the central core of the intact MRF does, indeed, normally have a powerful tonic desynchronizing influence on rhythmic EEG activity. But other brain stem centers appear to have a synchronizing influence on the frontal spindles, and can alter the cortical distribution of rhythmic activity when blocked in combination with MRF (fig. 2B).

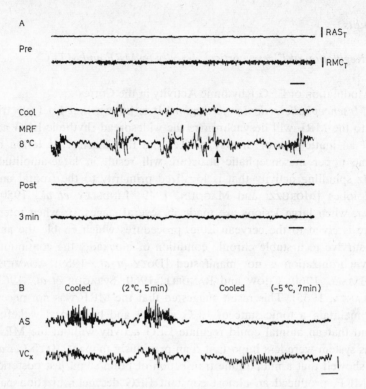

*Fig. 2.* Spontaneous spindles produced by bilateral cryogenic blockade in the mesencephalic reticular formation (MRF) of a chronic cat preparation. *A* Transcortical records from the anterior sigmoid (RAS$_T$) and far lateral anteroposterior sigmoid motor cortex (RMC$_T$) before (Pre), during (Cool MRF 8 °C), and 3 min after (Post) an extended 12-hour period of cryogenic blockade. A strong tail-pinch (arrow) was ineffective in producing behavioral arousal or persistent EEG desynchronization during the blockade. *B* Monopolar recordings from anterior sigmoid (AS) and primary visual cortex (VC$_X$) during moderate (2 °C) and intense (–5 °C) cooling of probes in the MRF. Note that the traces during the intense cooling, recorded only 2 min after the moderate cooling, manifest lack of synchronization in the frontal cortex, but not in the posterior areas. Calibrations: *A* 200 $\mu$V, 1 sec; *B* 100 $\mu$V, 1 sec; surface negative polarity, upward deflection. From SKINNER [1970a].

*b) Mediothalamic-frontocortical system.* DEMPSEY and MORISON [1942a, b] and MORISON and DEMPSEY [1942, 1943] found that midline thalamic stimulation at 8–12 Hz resulted in a series of monophasic negative cortical EPs that incremented in amplitude; such *recruiting responses* were found to be largest in the frontal half of the cortex. More lateral thalamic stimulation produced positive-negative cortical EPs which they called *augmenting responses*. Contrary to earlier suggestions, waveform criteria cannot distinguish between these types of responses since stimulation of any thalamic nucleus elicits positive-negative potentials in the known primary anatomical projection zone, while monophasic negative responses appear in surrounding areas. This distribution of potentials occurs whether a medial or a lateral thalamic nucleus is stimulated [SCHLAG and VILLABLANCA, 1967]. Our laboratory has nevertheless preferred to keep the terms recruiting and augmenting responses, even though they cannot be specified by waveform, for they can be defined by their effect on behavior. Mediothalamic stimulation, traditionally associated with recruiting responses, will completely disrupt ongoing behavior [MAHUT, 1964; BUSER *et al.*, 1964; BUCHWALD *et al.*, 1961] whereas slightly more lateral thalamic stimulation will not [PECCI-SAVAADRA *et al.*, 1965]. Thus, by our criteria, recruiting responses are elicited by mediothalamic stimuli, while augmenting responses are produced by stimulation of more lateral thalamic nuclei.

Blockade of the medial thalamus, the frontal granular cortex, or the bidirectional pathway interconnecting them (the inferior thalamic peduncle, ITP) will abolish recruiting responses and spontaneous spindle bursts that follow blockade of the MRF [VELASCO and LINDSLEY, 1965; SKINNER and LINDSLEY, 1967, 1971; VELASCO *et al.*, 1968; SKINNER, 1971b, c]. The augmenting responses, however, are unaffected by such blockade (fig. 3) [SKINNER and LINDSLEY, 1967; SKINNER, 1971b] as are certain components of synchronous activity induced by other means, such as by barbiturates, spontaneous sleep, etc. [SKINNER, 1971b]. These results show the specificity of the MTFCS in the regulation of only the type of cortical synchronization that is associated with recruiting responses.

After identifying the mediothalamic mechanism as the one underlying internal inhibition, MAGOUN [1963] conceived that the principle of reciprocal innervation (Sherrington) would appear relevant to the manner in which MRF and MTFCS determine the alternating patterns of brain activity. However, as will be shown below, this idea of reciprocal innervation holds only for the regulation of EEG synchronization and other bioelectric activities, but does not hold for the regulation of behavior.

## 2. Modulation of Sensory EP Amplitude in the Cortex

*a) Mesencephalic reticular formation.* Stimulation of the MRF will increase the amplitude of the visual EP produced by optic tract stimula-

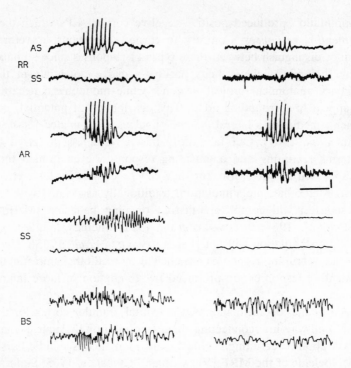

*Fig. 3.* Effects of small bilateral lesions in the ITP (right column) on several forms of EEG synchronization recorded (control, left column) in frontal (anterior sigmoid, As) and posterior (suprasylvian, SS) cortices. RR = Recruiting responses produced by 8 Hz stimulation of the medial thalamus (nu. centralis medialis); AR = augmenting responses produced by 8 Hz stimulation of the lateral thalamus (nu. ventralis lateralis) in the same chronic animals in which the RR was recorded; SS = spontaneous spindles produced by small bilateral lesions confined to the mesencephalic reticular formation; BS = barbiturate spindles produced by a 20-mg/kg dose of sodium pentobarbital. Note that the ITP lesions abolished RRs and SSs and some components of BSs without affecting ARs or other components of BSs. Calibrations: 100 μV, 1 sec; negative up.

tion and in a cerveau isolé the relative MRF facilitation is greater if produced during spindling episodes than during desynchronization intervals [BREMER and STOUPEL, 1959; DUMONT and DELL, 1960]. The latter result suggests that the enhancement of the VEP was perhaps suppressed by the spindling activity. ROSSI *et al.* [1965] showed that the amplitudes of VEPs during sleep were lower during EEG synchronization and higher during desynchronized sleep (i.e. rapid eye movement sleep or REMs.

However, CORDEAU et al. [1965] showed that during slow-wave sleep (SWS) the variability of the VEP amplitudes elicited from the optic tract was very high, manifesting not only the lowest amplitudes, but the largest as well. Any correlation between the amplitude of the synchronous EEG activity and the VEP is likely to be invalid unless the large variability factor is dealt with appropriately. Furthermore, sleep is certainly not a unitary process, and synchronization in one thalamocortical system does not mean that another system is necessarily manifesting synchronization at the same time. The site chosen for recording the synchronous activity may be very important when attempting to correlate its amplitude with that of a sensory EP.

*b) Mediothalamic-frontocortical system.* JASPER and AJMONE-MARSAN [1952] showed an inverse relationship between the amplitude of the recruiting response produced by thalamic stimulation in ventralis anterior and the primary EP to lateral geniculate stimulation. Thus, during activation of the MTFCS, the primary sensory EP appears to be reduced in amplitude. We found the same inverse correlation during blockade in the MTFCS [SKINNER and LINDSLEY, 1967] by cooling the ITP when the recruiting response gradually reduced in amplitude and the EP increased (fig. 4, 5).

In conclusion, the consequences of action of stimulation and lesion within the MRF are opposite to those within the MTFCS, not only for the regulation of EEG rhythmic activity, but also for the modulation of sensory EP amplitude. The closely coupled inverse relationship between the amplitude of the recruiting response (and other related forms of EEG rhythmic activity) and that of the sensory EP suggests a common mechanism regulating both types of bioelectric activity.

### 3. Modulation of Slow-Potential Shifts in the Cortex

*a) Mesencephalic reticular formation.* ARDUINI et al. [1957] first showed that a negative slow potential (SP) or DC shift could be produced in the frontal cortex by stimulation of various sensory nerves that project into the MRF or by stimulation of the MRF itself. At onset of sleep, presumably associated with a decrease in MRF activation, a surface-positive SP is recorded in the frontal cortex [CASPERS, 1963, 1965].

*b) Mediothalamic-frontocortical system.* GOLDRING and O'LEARY [1957] showed that low-frequency stimulation of the medial thalamus produces negative SP shifts in the baseline of the recruiting response of the frontal cortex. However, they also occasionally observed the recruit-

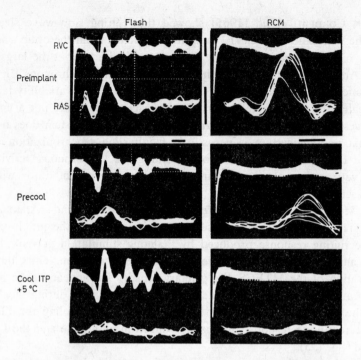

*Fig. 4.* Enhancement of photic-evoked responses and abolition of recruiting responses by blockade in the ITP. Photic stimuli (Flash) and 8 Hz thalamic stimuli (RCM = right center median, 0.5 mm from midline) were given to a Flaxedil-immobilized cat with dilated pupils. Responses were recorded monopolarly from the right primary visual cortex (RVC) and the right frontal anterior sigmoid cortex (RAS) before bilateral cryoprobes were implanted (preimplant), after implantation (i.e. slight surgical intervention) (Precool), and during cooling of probe tips to +5 °C (Cool ITP +5 °C). Note inverse relationship between the amplitude of the visual-evoked potentials and the recruiting responses. Calibrations: 100 µV, 20 msec; negative up. From SKINNER and LINDSLEY [1967].

ing responses to be superimposed upon a positive SP. We showed that more lateral low-frequency thalamic stimulation produced the negative cortical responses, whereas stimulation at the midline produced either the positive cortical response or none at all. Our present results confirm that, indeed, mediothalamic stimulation produces only positive SPs whereas laterothalamic stimulation in the rostral part of nu. ventralis lateralis (VL), adjacent to R produces the negative SPs. Stimulation in the center of VL has little or no effect on the SPs. It may be that the anterior VL stimuli

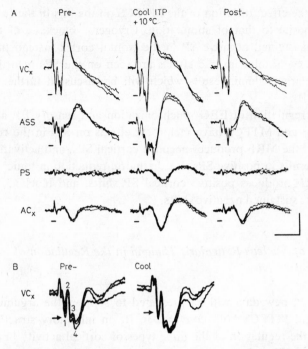

*Fig. 5.* Enhancement of VEPs at thalamic and cortical levels by cryogenic blockade of the ITP. *A* Responses elicited by optic radiation stimulation near the dorsolateral geniculate body were recorded ipsilaterally from the surface of primary visual cortex ($VC_X$), anterior suprasylvian association cortex (ASS), posterior-sigmoid association cortex (PS), and primary auditory nonprojection cortex ($AC_X$) before (Pre-), during (Cool ITP +10 °C), and 3 min after (Post-) the cryogenic blockade. The enhancement of the third and fourth positive peaks (identified in *B*, below) indicates a greater cortical response to a constant afferent input (peak 1 remains unchanged). *B* Response elicited by optic tract stimulation were recorded monopolarly from ipsilateral primary visual cortex. Note that the first positive peak, which represents the magnitude of the afferent input to the cortex, and the third and fourth peaks, which represent the cortical response to the input, are all enhanced by cooling the ITP (10 °C). Each trace is 30 averaged EPs. Calibrations: *A* 100 µV, 10 msec; *B* 100 µV, 5 msec; negative up. From SKINNER and LINDSLEY [1971].

actually activate the subthalamic fibers from the MRF that seem to project near or into the anterior pole of the thalamus [SCHEIBEL and SCHEIBEL, 1967; MILLHOUSE, 1969] and thereby produce the typical response elicited by direct MRF stimulation, namely cortical SPs that are negative in polarity.

In contrast, the effect of lesion of the MTFCS on the SPs in the frontal cortex is opposite to that of stimulation. Cryogenic blockade of the ITP produces a sustained negative SP in the frontal cortex instead of a positive one (fig. 6). Similar inverse effects are seen on the SPs recorded in nucleus reticularis thalami, results which will be discussed further in the next section (B).

As with the regulation of EEG synchronization and sensory EP amplitude, the MRF and MTFCS have reciprocal effects on SPs in the cortex. Activation of the MRF produces negative cortical SPs, and activation of the MTFCS results in positive SPs. Furthermore, reduction in tonic activity of the MRF produces positive cortical SP shifts, and blockade in the MTFCS elicits sustained negative shifts.

## B. The Role of Nucleus Reticularis Thalami in the Regulation of Electrocortical Activity

In this section, new data will be presented to support the argument that the MRF and MTFCS both converge in R, an inhibitory structure that is crucial in the regulation of the three types of cortical activity [YINGLING and SKINNER, this volume].

### 1. Anatomical Structure of Nu. Reticularis Thalami

*a) Output from R cells.* The thalamic reticular nucleus develops embryologically from the ventral thalamus and migrates dorsally to envelop most of the outer surface of the sensory and association nuclei of the dorsal thalamus [ROSE, 1952]. By making ablations in the cortex and then observing degenerative changes in R, ROSE [1952] interpreted that the axons of R project to the cortex and that the degeneration he observed was retrograde. However, he cautiously pointed out that if the axons of R projected back into thalamic nuclei which were degenerating due to the cortical ablation, then the degeneration in R could be caused by transneuronal processes. The latter interpretation was in line with the Golgi studies of RAMÓN Y CAJAL [1911] which suggested that the axons from R cells projected back into the thalamus rather than toward the cortex. However, an anatomical system over which widespread recruiting responses could be transmitted was eagerly being sought in the fifties. SCHEIBEL and SCHEIBEL [1966] finally did the definitive study of R, using Golgi-stained material, and showed that most, if not all, axons from R project back into the thalamus and not to the cortex. Furthermore, they showed that R cells had highly bifurcated axons and seemed to project back into the thalamic nucleus that innervated them, as well as diffusely to other thalamic regions. These observations have recently been confirmed by JONES [1975] using tritium-labeled amino acids to make autoradiographs.

*b) Input to R cells.* Approximately 10% of the thalamocortical and cortico-thalamic fibres project collaterals into R as they pass through it [SCHEIBEL and SCHEIBEL, personal commun.]. In the rostral region of R (i.e. $R_{VA}$), but not in the rest of the structure, a dense neuropil occurs in which major inputs also arise from the mesencephalic reticular formation, the medial thalamus, and the frontal granular cortex [SCHEIBEL and SCHEIBEL, 1966; 1972]. There are also inputs from the caudate nucleus and the anterior limb of the internal capsule via collateral branches from axons projecting into the thalamus, especially into ventralis anterior [SCHEIBEL and SCHEIBEL, 1966]. It is interesting that all or most of the inputs into R cells from other structures are via axon collaterals of fibers that penetrate the nucleus in their projection to or from the thalamus.

2. Inhibitory and Excitatory Slow Potentials Produced in R

Stimulation of the MTFCS and MRF at their optimum frequencies produces fronto*cortical* SPs of opposite polarity, as discussed above; concurrently, very large amplitude potentials (5–15 mV) are produced in R that are of opposite polarity to the cortical SPs. Low-frequency stimulation of the medial thalamus (NCM) produces in the frontal cortex (AS) monophasic negative recruiting responses superimposed upon surface-positive SPs and in R monophasic positive recruiting responses superimposed upon negative SPs (fig. 6A). High-frequency stimulation of the MRF produces opposite polarity SP responses in both locations (fig. 6B). Neither medial thalamic (NCM, CM, VA) nor lateral thalamic (VL, VPL, LGN) nuclei manifested the giant subcortical SPs that were recorded exclusively in R in the chronic preparations, although exhaustive thalamic investigations were not performed.

Recording from single units in R while stimulating the medial thalamus or MRF to evoke SPs revealed complete silence of the unit during positive shifts in R and driving of the unit during negative SPs in R [YINGLING and SKINNER, this volume]. Long duration membrane potential shifts have been recorded intracellularly in R cells during the spontaneous regulation of their action potentials [WASZAK, 1973, 1974], a finding which suggests that the electrogenesis of the extracellular SPs is related to

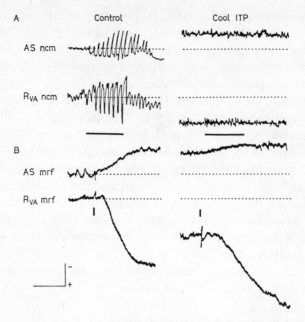

*Fig. 6.* SP shifts produced by stimulation of the medial thalamus and mesencephalic reticular formation and by cryogenic blockade in the ITP. *A* Stimulation (8 Hz, dark line) of nucleus centralis medialis (NCM) produces monophasic negative recruiting responses (RRs), superimposed upon positive SP shifts, which are recorded from the surface of the anterior sigmoid cortex (AS); monophasic positive RRs, superimposed upon a negative SP shift, are simultaneously recorded from nucleus reticularis thalami ($R_{VA}$). Cryogenic blockade of the ITP (Cool ITP) abolishes both the RRs and SPs and produces a sustained negative potential on the AS and a constant positive potential in R. *B* Brief stimulation (250 msec, 250 Hz) of the mesencephalic reticular formation (mrf) produces surface-negative SPs on the AS and positive SPs in R. Cryogenic blockade (Cool ITP) abolishes the SP shift in AS but not in R. All responses are from a single chronic cat preparation. Calibrations: *A* 500 $\mu$V, 1 sec; *B* 1,000 $\mu$V, 10 sec; negative up. From SKINNER and YINGLING [1976].

these tonic postsynaptic potentials in R cells. Stimulation of the MRF results in the immediate inhibition of unit discharges in $R_{VA}$ (fig. 5 in the following paper), whereas the onset and peak latencies of the associated positive SP shift are in the order of seconds (fig. 7 and 8 in the following paper). If the excitability of the units is related to the same process reflected by the SP, then why are the latencies of the two types of responses so different in time? SOMJEN and co-workers [LOTHMAN and SOMJEN,

1975; LOTHMAN et al., 1975] have recently hypothesized that a syncytium of glial cells interconnected by low-resistance gap junctions produces the separation of charge that results in the recorded SPs. These glial cells appear to respond to local shifts in the extracellular potassium ion concentrations associated with the depolarization or hyperpolarization of the adjacent neurons. Hence, the offset in time between the neural unit activity and the glial SP response could be due either to the potassium diffusion time in the extracellular space or to a slow response process of the glial cell membrane to the activity in the adjacent neurons.

MTFCS and MRF independently regulate the activity in R cells since the SP response in R to MRF stimulation persists after blocking the MTFCS (fig. 6, cool ITP). This result suggests that inputs from both the MRF and the MTFCS converge upon R and are integrated there, a finding which is consistent with the anatomical observations. Note that ITP cooling produces surface-negative shifts in the cortex and positive shifts in R, potentials which are opposite in polarity to those produced by mediothalamic stimulation.

### 3. Synchronous Activity Mediated by R

Since ANDERSEN and ECCLES [1962] and PURPURA and COHEN [1962] first noted that long-duration IPSPs in thalamic cells are associated with spontaneous spindles and recruiting responses, it has been interpreted that the origin of these thalamic IPSPs was the basic element underlying cortical synchronization. The isolated thalamus is capable of synchronization [VILLABLANCA and SCHLAG, 1968], a finding which suggests that at least some of the timing elements are subcortical. The isolated cortex is quiescent unless low-frequency stimulation of the white matter occurs, in which case incremental responses resembling recruiting responses are elicited [SCHLAG and VILLABLANCA, 1967]. The question then arises as to the location of the subcortical inhibitory cells that underlie the generation of the cortical synchronous activity.

SCHLAG and WASZAK [1970, 1971] have shown that during either spontaneous or electrically elicited synchronization, R cells manifest 200- to 400-Hz bursts of activity that are associated with the occurrence of IPSPs in the thalamic cells. However, cellular groups other than R also appear to give rise to IPSPs in the thalamus [ANDERSEN et al., 1964]. It may well be that there are different inhibitory mechanisms responsible for augmenting and recruiting responses, for ITP blockade abolishes recruiting responses and spontaneous spindles without affecting augmenting re-

Control                                              Les ITP

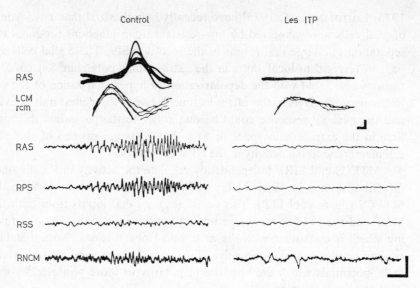

RAS

LCM
rcm

RAS

RPS

RSS

RNCM

*Fig. 7.* Abolition of cortical and thalamic recruiting responses and spontaneous spindles by bilateral lesions in the ITP. Upper oscilloscope records: Stimulation
(8 Hz) of the right center median nucleus (rcm) produces recruiting responses in
the right anterior sigmoid cortex (RAS) and left center median (LCM) that were
totally abolished following the lesions (Les ITP). Lower inkwriter traces: Bilateral
lesions of the MRF resulted in large-amplitude spontaneous spindles recorded in the
right anterior sigmoid cortex (RAS), right posterior sigmoid cortex (RPS), and right
nucleus centralis medialis (RNCM), but not in the right suprasylvian cortex (RSS).
The synchronous activity was abolished following the lesions in the ITP. Flaxedil-
immobilized cat. Calibrations: 100 μV, 10 msec (upper); 100 μV, 1 sec (lower);
negative up, monopolar recordings.

sponses (fig. 3). Furthermore, the ITP cooling or lesions abolish the thal-
amically induced responses in the thalamus as well as in the cortex
(fig. 7), a finding which implies that a wholly thalamic mechanism cannot
explain the generation of the recruiting type of synchronous activity. With
total ablation of the cortex, a spontaneous form of synchronization is restored in the thalamus [SCHLAG and VILLABLANCA, 1967] but it is not
known whether the R cells then disclose their bursting of unit activity or
if other cellular groups become active. During ITP blockade, the R units
are no longer capable of being driven by medial thalamic stimuli, a finding which suggests that their activation is necessary for the generation of
the recruiting type of synchronization [YINGLING and SKINNER, this vol-
ume].

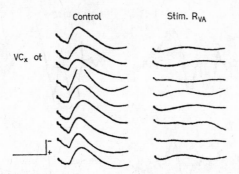

Fig. 8. Blockade of EPs by stimulation in the anterior neuropil region of nucleus reticularis thalami ($R_{VA}$). Stimulation of the optic tract (ot) produced VEPs in the primary visual cortex ($VC_X$) that were totally abolished by a conditioning stimulus (50 msec, 150 Hz) in $R_{VA}$, delivered 150 msec preceding the ot stimulus (Stim. $R_{VA}$). Chronic cat preparation. Calibrations: 400 $\mu$V, 10 msec. From SKINNER and YINGLING [1976].

## 4. EP Modulation by R

Figure 8 shows the effects of stimulation in the anterior neuropil region of R on a primary VEP to optic-tract (OT) stimulation. High frequency (100 Hz) stimulation of the $R_{VA}$ electrode in this chronic preparation resulted in total suppression of the VEP 1–150 msec after the conditioning train, a finding which suggests complete block at the thalamic level. Stimulation of critical loci in other regions of R reliably produced inhibitory effects on other sensory signals, there being a modality-specific organization in R [YINGLING and SKINNER, this volume]. Topographical organization of sense modality also appears to exist in the MTFCS. Bilateral cryoprobes placed symmetrically in a given region of the ITP (fig. 9) when cooled to 15 °C enhanced VEPs, but did not affect auditory EPs (AEP). However, increasing the magnitude of the blockade in the ITP by cooling to 10 °C enhanced both the VEPs and AEPs. Some, if not all, of the descending ITP fibers project upon $R_{VA}$ cells in the anterior neuropil region. Interconnections then are made between the anterior R cells and the more posterior ones apparently via long dendritic bundles as described by SCHEIBEL and SCHEIBEL [1972]. In conclusion, the modality-specificity that is inherent in the MTFCS appears to be maintained within the system upon which it projects.

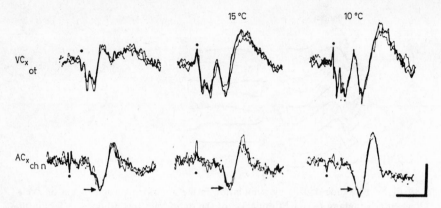

*Fig. 9.* Topographical organization of sense modalities in the ITP. Independent enhancement of visual and auditory EPs occurred during two levels of cryogenic blockade in the ITP. Cooling to 15 °C increased VEPs but not AEPs (middle column) and cooling to 10 °C enhanced both (right). VEPs were recorded in primary cortex (VC$_X$) and elicited by optic tract (ot) stimulation. AEPs were recorded in primary cortex (AC$_X$) and produced by dorsal cochlear nucleus stimulation (ch n). Each trace represents 30 averaged responses, all recorded from the same chronic cat preparation. Calibrations: 200 $\mu$V, 10 msec; negative up, monopolar recordings. From SKINNER and LINDSLEY [1971].

## C. Behavioral Analysis of the MTFCS and MRF

### 1. Inability to Inhibit Strong Response Tendencies

At the 1964 International Symposium on the frontal granular cortex and behavior, an interpretation that seemed to fit most data was the suggestion that the animal with lesions in the frontal lobe is unable to inhibit a strong response tendency [KONORSKI and LAWICKA, 1964; BRUTKOWSKI, 1964; MISHKIN, 1964]. Thus, a monkey with frontal lesions, when required to change its bar-press behavior from the previously correct stimulus to the previously incorrect one, persisted in responding to the previously reinforced stimulus. However, if the previously incorrect stimulus was replaced with a novel stimulus, the animals then shifted their responses normally, i.e. a competing strong response tendency towards novel stimuli compensated for the strong response tendency produced by the previous reinforcement [MISHKIN, 1964]. These and other experiments show that if the experimenter structures the stimulus environment so as to compensate for the strong response tendencies of subjects with frontal lobe lesions, then the behavioral deficit is not manifested. Thus, the function of

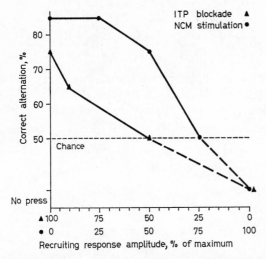

*Fig. 10.* Medial thalamic stimulation (8 Hz) and cryogenic blockade of the ITP have the *same* effect on reducing performance of a single-alternation task. Increasing the intensity of stimulation of nucleus centralis medialis (NCM) increases recruiting responses and reduces percent correct performance; increasing ITP blockade, which will reduce test recruiting responses proportionally, also reduces performance. Percent correct alternation has been plotted as a function of the percent increase or decrease in the maximum amplitude of the recruiting response. Each point represents the average of three animals, and all are statistically significantly different (p<0.05) from each other, except for the 0 and 25% recruiting response amplitude points on the NCM stimulation curve.

the intact frontal lobes is to provide this response control toward the particular stimuli.

MRF and MTFCS do not have similar but opposite effects on behavior as they do on EPs. The inability to inhibit a strong response tendency that is produced by lesions in the MTFCS is quite different from the arousal and alerting behavior produced by MRF stimulation. Moreover, lesion compared to stimulation within the MTFCS does not produce opposite effects on behavior, but rather they both produce the *same* effect, as illustrated by figure 10. In contrast, increments in stimulation and blockade in the MRF have opposite effects on the spectrum of vigilance behaviors that the MRF regulates. Although the MRF and MTFCS each regulate cortical synchronization and EP amplitude, they clearly mediate different processes and therefore are not simply excitatory and inihibitory structures reciprocally interconnected to modulate a unitary process, as a simplistic interpretation would imply.

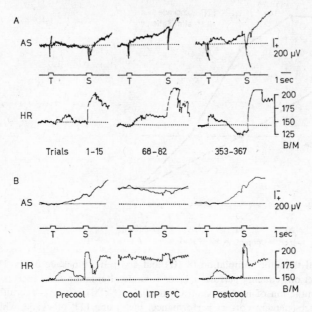

*Fig. 11.* Abolition of both the conditioned SP in the AS and the HR during cryogenic blockade in the ITP. The responses, which occurred during acquisition of tone (T)-shock (S) conditioning, are shown in *A*. Note parallel changes in the waveform of the response during each phase of conditioning. After overconditioning (1,000 trials), the responses changed further, as shown in *B* (Pre cool). Cooling the ITP to 5 °C abolished both the SP and the cardiac responses, but changed the baselines of each. 15 responses were averaged for each trace. AS records are transcortical, surface-negative up; HR traces are calibrated in beats per min (B/M).

## 2. Classical Conditioning

Figure 11A shows the acquisition of a classically conditioned slow potential response recorded in the AS and a conditioned rate response recorded from the heart (HR). A tone-shock paradigm was used in which a 0.5-sec tone forewarned a mild electric shock to the hind limbs (50 V, 100 Hz, 0.5-msec pulse duration, 0.5-sec train) that was delivered 4 sec later. Each block is representative of initial (1–15), early (68–82), and late (353–367) phase of conditioning for five chronic cat preparations that showed essentially similar responses, but varied in the number of trials necessary to reach each phase. The responses recorded during the interstimulus interval of the initial 15 trials did not differ from the records fol-

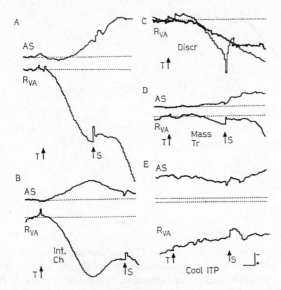

*Fig. 12.* SP responses recorded from the frontal cortex (AS) and nucleus reticularis thalami ($R_{VA}$) during a tone (T)-shock (S) conditioning paradigm. *A* Responses after overconditioning. *B* Responses immediately after changing interstimulus interval from 4 to 6 sec (Int Ch). *C* Reduction in SP amplitude to a nonreinforced tone of higher frequency (thicker trace), randomly interspersed between the reinforced tones (thinner trace) in a discrimination paradigm (Discr). *D* Responses after changing intertrial intervals from 3.0+1.5 min to 30+15 sec (Mass Tr). *E* Responses after bilateral cryogenic blockade of the ITP (Cool ITP). Expectancy, selective perception, and habituation are all reflected in these SP responses (*B, C,* and *D,* respectively). The integrity of the ITP is necessary for their manifestation *(E).* Each trace is the average of 15 responses. Calibrations: 200 $\mu$V, 1 sec. From SKINNER and YINGLING [1976].

lowing the presentation of the tone alone. The changes in conditioned frontal cortex SPs during acquisition are seen to be closely correlated with the changes in the conditioned cardiac responses. The phase of overconditioning (1,000 trials or more) is shown in the left-hand records of figure 11B for a different cat. Cryogenic blockade of the ITP, sufficient to abolish recruiting responses, also abolished both the frontal cortex SPs and the cardiac-conditioned responses, but the conditioned behavioral components were unaffected. The tone continued to evoke an orienting reaction of the ears towards the speaker, followed by a stereotyped crouching movement just preceding the negative shock reinforcement.

Figure 12 shows that conditioned SP responses, recorded simultane-

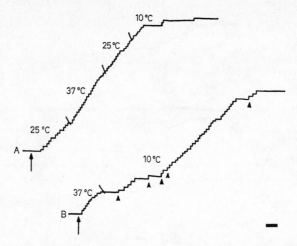

*Fig. 13.* Effects of cryogenic blockade in the ITP on bar-press rate. *A* Cryoprobes were cooled bilaterally to the temperatures shown while the animals barpressed for a milk reward, as illustrated by the cumulative response records. *B* After cooling to 10 °C, the animal was 'coaxed' back to the bar by free rewards (triangles), but would often turn away from the bar spontaneously without such free rewards. Calibrations: Each step on the ordinate is one bar-press; time mark for the abscissa is 1 sec. From Skinner and Lindsley [1967].

ously from both AS and from R, manifested temporal conditioning to the interstimulus interval (fig. 12B), discrimination of the conditioned stimulus (fig. 12C), and response decrement during massed trials (fig. 12D), phenomena that are all characteristic of classically conditioned behavioral responses. During all of these situations depicted in figure 12, blockade of the MTFCS at the level of the ITP abolished the SPs without affecting the manifestation of the overt behavioral components. In a sensory-sensory conditioning paradigm, a great deal of cerebral activity occurs that is disassociated from the simple behavioral components of the *already established* conditioned response. In two additional naive animals tested, no signs of acquisition of the tone-shock conditioned response occurred after the first 200 trials had been given *during* ITP blockade. Thus, the integrity of the ITP is necessary for the learning to occur, but once acquisition is complete, the overt behavioral components seem to be mediated independently of the MTFCS. In order to understand better the role of the ITP in behavior, the performance of the animal during ITP blockade in more complex behavioral tasks must be examined.

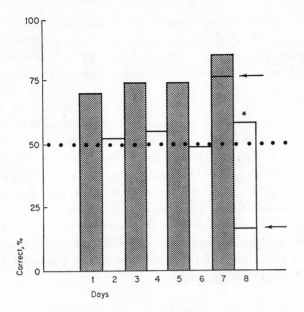

*Fig. 14.* Deficits in performance of a single-alternation task during partial cryogenic blockade of the ITP. Each vertical bar represents the mean percent correct
scores for the group of five animals during control levels of cooling to 25 °C (shad-
ed bars) and during ITP-blocking levels of cooling to 15 °C (unshaded bars). Each
animal was experimented upon for 8 consecutive days, alternating the cooling temperatures. By the 7th and 8th days, the animals had developed a habit of leaving a
paw outstretched on the bar just pressed, a strategy that occurred in approximately
half of the trials. The performance levels on *nonstrategy* trials (arrows) was less
than chance during 15 °C cooling, a finding that indicates perseveration of responding to the last reinforced bar. From SKINNER and LINDSLEY [1967].

### 3. Operant Conditioning

Figure 13 shows that ITP blockade, sufficient to abolish recruiting
responses (10 °C), disrupts the maintenance of performance of a simple
bar-press task. By attracting the animal back to the bar with free rewards
(triangles), the animal could be 'coaxed' to bar-press for limited periods
but always turned away from the bar spontaneously to groom, to sniff the
floor, or to look out the window. While wandering around in the bar-
press chamber, the animal would encounter the bar by chance and then
bar-press a few times before once again turning away and pursuing other
activities.

Figure 14 shows that moderate cryogenic blockade, insufficient to cause bar-pressing to cease, but sufficient to reduce recruiting responses and enhance optic tract elicited VEPs, prevents the correct performance of a single alternation bar-press task. When analysis of bar-press trials was made on days 7 and 8, it was found that during approximately one half of the trials, all the animals used the strategy of leaving one paw outstretched on the lever that was just pressed while drinking the milk reward from a center food cup. They then made a correct response during the next trial. However, if their ITP was partially blocked when non-strategy responses occurred, then the animals tended to press again the bar just pressed if their ITP was partially blocked (day 8, arrow); if ITP cooling was insufficient to affect recruiting responses or visual EPs then the animals responded normally (day 7, arrows). This perseveration of responding to the last reinforced bar during ITP blockade was independent of whether a left or a right bar had previously been pressed. Thus, in operant conditioning the integrity of the MTFCS is necessary in order for the overt behavioral act to be manifested.

## Discussion

### A. Emergence of a Neurophysiological Model of Attention Based on Physiological and Behavioral Analysis

#### 1. Distinct Behavioral Functions of the MTFCS and MRF

The MTFCS and MRF can each regulate independently the three types of bioelectric activities that have been associated with defined states of attention, namely synchronous EEG, sensory EPs, and SP shifts. The regulation appears to result from excitation by the MTFCS and inhibition by the MRF on the cells of R, a structure which has inhibitory control over the transmission through the sensory relay nuclei. A simplistic model, while seemingly appropriate to summarize the reciprocal effects of the MRF and MTFCS on the three types of bioelectric activities, failed to account for the behavioral effects. For example, stimulation compared to lesion within the MRF did produce opposite effects on behavior, but stimulation and lesion within the MTFCS resulted in the *same* behavioral changes. Furthermore, the effect of stimulation of the MRF (behavioral alerting and arousal) was quite different from that produced by lesion of the MTFCS (inability to perform a single alternation task), though both procedures did result in similar changes in cortical EPs.

Stimulation or neural blockade in the MRF increases or decreases its output and, depending upon the particular *level of activation* that results from such procedures, there occurs a unique shift in behavior to one of many possible points along a linear spectrum from comatose to highly active. Turning on the sensory gates by a strong activation of the MRF has the opposite consequence on behavior as turning them all off. By contrast, stimulation or lesion in the MTFCS produces the same type of change in behavior, a finding which suggests that a critical *pattern of activation* in the MTFCS (not just a level of activation) is essential to regulate behavior. Thus, the two systems subserve distinct behavioral functions and are not simply reciprocally operating components of the same system, as previously thought.

## 2. Selective versus General Regulation of Evoked Potentials

Discrete anatomical organization is apparent within the MTFCS, as evidenced by the independent visual and auditory EP changes during progressive functional blockade of the ITP. The modality-specific organization also appears in R, the inhibitory system through which the MTFCS exerts its effects upon the sensory systems [YINGLING and SKINNER, this volume]. Such evidence for modality-specific organization is completely lacking for the MRF which has a diffuse, widespread, generalized organization [JASPER, 1960; LINDSLEY, 1960]. Another contrast between the two systems is that the effects of MTFCS activation on the various EPs seem to return to the baseline condition very rapidly, whereas the effects of even brief MRF stimulation persists for 20–30 sec. This phasic versus tonic character of the two systems has been noted before [cf. JASPER, 1960].

In conclusion, our interpretation of MTFCS function is that it selectively regulates the three types of bioelectric activity because it operates as a *specifically* organized system with *phasic* control. The MRF, on the other hand, maintains a level of activation in a diffusely organized system that underlies *tonic* changes, characteristics which are all more easily associated with a generalized regulatory process.

## 3. Selective Inhibition of Irrelevant Stimuli

Blockade of the MTFCS elicits a specific behavioral deficit. The animal can no longer inhibit any strong tendency to respond, either to relevant or irrelevant stimuli, and because of this can no longer maintain its performance in an operantly conditioned task. The animal is still capable, however, of simple bar-pressing and continues to manifest normal primitive behaviors (eating, grooming, walking), orienting reactions, and certain overt behavioral components of the aversive conditioned response. This shows that the behavioral elements of either the operant or classical conditioned response appear to remain intact while the ability to regulate these responses is lost during disruption of MTFCS function. If the experimenter changes the significance of the stimulus environment, for example, by introducing a novel positive stimulus at the time of reversal in a discrimination-reversal task [MISHKIN, 1964], then compensation for the deficit can occur. This suggests that the MTFCS, similar to the intervening experimenter, normally controls the significance of some features of the stimulus environment in such a way that irrelevant responses are suppressed.

The frontal lobe damaged or ITP-blocked animal is unable not only to direct or maintain his attention but also to suppress the transmission to the cortex of activity evoked by a repetitious and irrelevant stimulus. This latter point is illustrated by the enhancement of the irrelevant auditory and visual EPs in the cortex during ITP blockade or lesion of the frontal cortex. Thus, the ability of the intact animal to focus its attention occurs by way of inhibition in the thalamocortical circuits carrying *irrelevant* information. This result implies that selective attention emerges via selective inhibition in certain sensory channels that the animal must *know in advance* are irrelevant to its situation. How this prior knowledge is obtained is not known, but its acquisition may be related to the subsidence of the orienting reaction.

LURIA and HOMSKAYA [1970] have attributed the deficit following frontal lobe lesions to an intensification of, or inability to inhibit, orienting reactions. It appears that the subject with a blocked MTFCS no longer has the ability to manifest *rapid* behavioral habituation to a stimulus that initially produces an orienting reaction. Such a mechanism does not preclude the ability of other intact mechanisms to mediate a slower mechanism of habituation, for the frontal lobe lesioned animal is still capable of manifesting extinction of responses [KONORSKI and LAWICKA, 1964]. The events underlying the orienting reactions presumably are initiated at the brain stem level since MRF lesions render the animals comatose and therefore incapable of responding to stimuli. The function of the MTFCS appears to keep the orienting reactions under control by selectively inhibiting the ascent of sensory stimuli that are deemed by it to be irrelevant.

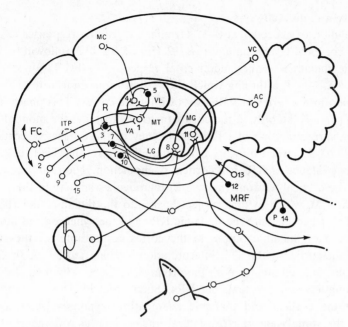

*Fig. 15.* Neural model for the gating of sensory relay nuclei in the thalamus. Inhibitory neurons are black, and excitatory ones are white. Both the FC and the MRF converge upon and regulate the pattern of activity in the cells in R. The R cells then provide inhibitory control over the thalamic relay nuclei (LG = lateral geniculate; MG = medial geniculate). AC = Auditory cortex; ITP = inferior thalamic peduncle; MC = motor cortex; MT = medial thalamus; P = pontine reticular formation; VA = nucleus ventralis anterior; VC = visual cortex; VL = nucleus ventralis lateralis.

## B. A Specific Neural Model for Selective Attention and General Arousal Based upon EP Analysis

Figure 15 shows the features of the model that can be supported from the present results. The neurons whose somas are white are excitatory and those with black somas are inhibitory. The cells in R may actually be excitatory chains of interneurons with an inhibitory neuron at their terminations. R is shown as having a thick anterior neuropil and enlargement adjacent to the geniculate bodies. The term evoked potential is meant in its broadest sense to include all three types of evoked bioelectric activity presented in the results.

## 1. Synchronous Activity

Stimulation of neuron 1 at 8–12 Hz elicits recruiting responses (RRs) in frontal cortex (FC). Stimulation (8–12 Hz) of the ITP following ablation of the thalamus evokes incremental responses in FC [SCHLAG and VILLABLANCA, 1967], a finding which shows that a mechanism for EP incrementation in the series of RRs exists within the cortex. This phasic RR excitation spreads laterally in the cortex (arrows), forming the monophasic negative surround zone of RRs. The latency of these negative cortical RRs is still 20–30 msec following ITP stimulation, a result which suggests that the long latency of RRs is a cortical phenomenon. The resultant activation of the cortical neurons (neuron 2) then evokes activity in the units in R (neuron 3), which in turn project back into the thalamus the IPSPs that are thought to mediate the thalamic RRs and the synchronized burst-pause pattern of thalamic output to the cortex responsible for the generation of the cortical RRs. This interpretation is supported by the finding that ITP blockade eliminates both the driving of neuron 3 by medial thalamic stimulation and the thalamic RRs. Such blockade, however, does not affect the cortical and thalamic augmenting responses (ARs) produced by the stimulation of more lateral nuclei, such as VL (neuron 4). Thus, the inhibitory interneurons that mediate the ARs appear to be elsewhere than in R, probably as suggested [ANDERSEN and SEARS, 1964] within the lateral thalamic nucleus itself (neuron 5).

Long-latency (15–40 msec) IPSPs occur in VL cells following 8–12 Hz stimulation of the medial thalamus (MT) [PURPURA and COHEN, 1962] and short-latency (1.5–4 msec) IPSPs occur in MT cells following VL stimulation [DESIRAJU and PURPURA, 1970]. The long-latency thalamic responses are apparently due to the delay encountered in the cortex prior to the activation of the R units, whereas the short-latency responses are quickly transmitted throughout the thalamus probably by intrinsic thalamic interneurons. The medial and lateral thalamic interconnections described suggest that the recruiting and augmenting response mechanisms can affect the synchronous activity in each other (note collateral axons of inhibitory neurons 3 and 5). These two types of intrathalamic inhibitory connections could explain why widespread thalamic spindles following MRF lesions are abolished by ITP blockade, but return following complete isolation of the thalamus from the cortex. For example, ITP blockade in the MRF-lesioned animal will abolish the thalamic spindles, but will not affect ARs, a result which suggests that the thalamus could support another type of synchronous activity during this condition, but somehow it is inhibited.

Following complete decortication, this inhibition is released and thalamic spindles reoccur.

The duality of the thalamic mechanisms for synchronization can also explain why other laboratories found forms of EEG synchronization that are not blocked following frontal lobe ablations. For example, the augmenting responses are found to be unaffected by ITP blockade or frontal lobe lesions, whereas the frontally projecting EEG spindles and recruiting responses are affected [SKINNER, 1971b]. ROBERTSON and LYNCH [1971] showed that large lesions in the vicinity of the MRF resulted in spindles in the posterior cortices (marginal and suprasylvian gyri) that were not abolished by frontal lobotomy. However, as can be seen in figure 7, small lesions confined to the core of the MRF result in only frontal spindles with no slow activity in the suprasylvian cortex. The spread of large lesions centered in the MRF are shown in figure 2B to abolish the frontal spindles, but leave slow activity unaffected in the posterior cortices, a finding which suggests that the synchronous activity produced by ROBERTSON and LYNCH was not that mediated exclusively by the MTFCS, and hence frontal lobotomies would not be expected to affect this type of cortical activity. A similar argument can be made for barbiturate-induced synchronization, because pentobarbital has a diffuse effect on brain stem mechanisms and results in massive synchronization in both frontal and posterior cortices. Certainly not all forms of synchronization in the suprasylvian cortex are abolished following frontal lobotomies [ROBERTSON and LYNCH, 1971; DAHL et al., 1972], but certain large-amplitude components are eliminated following ITP blockade (fig. 3) [SKINNER, 1971b].

Similarly, the type of incremental responses produced in the suprasylvian cortex by intralaminar thalamic stimulation, with electrodes situated between the medial and lateral thalamic nuclei, is also unaffected by frontal lobotomies [STAUNTON and SASAKI, 1971], because the synchronous activity in the posterior cortex results from the activation of lateral thalamic mechanisms. Pure recruiting responses produced by medial thalamic stimulation do not appear in the suprasylvian cortices (fig. 3).

The apparent, but unnecessary, controversy between the above-mentioned reports and those of our laboratory illustrate the problems involved when synchronous activity is defined by *waveform* rather than by the system that mediates it. All the above papers are actually in line with our own results that show MTFCS blockade does not abolish augmenting responses [SKINNER and LINDSLEY, 1967; SKINNER, 1971b].

## 2. Sensory Evoked Potentials

Activation of particular R cells by direct stimulation (neuron 7 and 10) results in complete suppression of sensory EPs mediated via thalamic relay nuclei (neurons 8 and 11). Regulation of these R cells apparently is mediated normally by FC cells (neurons 6 and 9) because ITP cooling, which blocks the fronto-R projections, leads to facilitated transmission through the sensory relay nuclei. Topographical organization of these regulatory elements exists within the ITP and small cryogenic blockade will affect only one modality (i.e. neurons 6, 7, and 8) without affecting another (i.e. neurons 9, 10, and 11). By increasing the size of the functional blockade in ITP, the latter system is also affected. This result indicates that the FC can exert a selective regulation of EP amplitude as opposed to a general regulation.

Inhibition of the R cells can be achieved by stimulation anywhere in the MRF (neuron 12) [YINGLING and SKINNER, this volume] and this results in a general facilitation of transmission through the relay nuclei. PURPURA et al. [1966] have shown that MRF stimulation not only abolishes IPSPs in thalamic relay cells, but also produces EPSPs. This latter effect is probably mediated by a more direct route (neuron 13). The MRF-R mechanism of general disinhibition of sensory relay nuclei may explain the general facilitating factor present during the conditioned emotional response situation in which a general increase in sensory EPs occurs in response to the highly arousing signal that warns the subject of an imminent shock [MARK and HALL, 1967]. Our model, in which the MRF and MTFCS converge at R, can explain how both selective and general regulation of the same sensory EP can occur.

## 3. Slow Potentials

Stimulation of the MRF (neuron 12) not only causes unit activity in R cells to cease, but simultaneously produces in R a very large SP shift of positive polarity, a response which is presumably associated with hyperpolarisations of R cell membranes. In FC, a surface-negative, depth-positive SP is also produced following the MRF stimulation, but only if the ITP is intact. Since R cells project only back into the thalamus, and sance one of the major projections of R is back into the MT, which in turn projects to FC via the ITP [SCHEIBEL and SCHEIBEL, 1966, 1967], it would appear that neuron 1 is a primary candidate for eliciting SPs in FC. Such a mechanism indicates that the MRF-evoked SPs in FC are the result of the removal of inhibition on neuron 1 by inhibition of neuron 3.

Stimulation of MT neurons (8–12 Hz) results in burst-pause activation of MT, VL, FC, and R cells. During one evoked burst-pause cycle of MT cells, there occurs in R approximately 20 msec after the stimulus, a positive RR that is superimposed upon a negative SP shift. The SP is accompanied by the increased firing of R units, a finding suggesting that the SP represents membrane depolarization. This interpretation is supported by an observation by WASZAK [1974] who found a tonic depolarizing shift in the membrane potential of R cells during a tripped spindle burst following single and double shocks to the vicinity of the intralaminar region of the thalamus. The positive RRs are thought to be superimposed upon the negative SPs in R, and not generated by the same process, because the positive RRs can be recorded in many parts of the thalamus and internal capsule, whereas the SP is confined to the vicinity of R. The electrogenesis of the SPs recorded in R and elsewhere is unknown, though some evidence suggests that glial cells may play a passive role in mediating them [CASTELLUCCI and GOLDRING, 1970; GROSSMAN and ROSMAN, 1971; LOTHMAN and SOMJEN, 1975].

During ITP blockade, a constant positive SP shift occurs in R, and both the previously evoked SPs and the superimposed RRs are totally abolished (fig. 6). This effect of ITP blockade on the SPs recorded in R suggests that, in order for RRs to be generated, a depolarizing influence from FC cells (neuron 2) upon R neurons (neuron 3) must be maintained. This must also be the case even if MT cells (neuron 1) are able to drive R cells (neuron 3) directly via an axon collateral. The present results cannot distinguish whether the failure of MT cells to drive R units is due to the failure of EPSPs from MT axon collaterals to reach the critical firing level or the failure of EPSPs to be generated by FC cells. What is clear is that ITP blockade causes positive SP shifts in R, a finding which suggests that R cell membranes hyperpolarize and thus prevent either possible source of EPSPs from driving the units.

## C. Extension of the Model:
## Regulation of the Autonomic Nervous System

Blockade of the ITP not only abolishes RRs and SP shifts and enhances EPs to irrelevant stimuli, but also eliminates the cardiac-conditioned response to a tone reinforced by an aversive shock. Frontal lobe ablations have also been shown to abolish this response [SMITH et al.,

1968]. Anatomical evidence for projections from the orbitofrontal cortex into the hypothalamus, subthalamus, and tegmentum [NAUTA, 1964; MILLHOUSE, 1969] illustrates the high degree of connectivity of the cortical component of the MTFCS with known cardiovascular regulatory structures (neuron 15 in fig. 15). A recent review of the neural control of the heart and circulation [SMITH, 1974] pointed out that higher brain structures control cardiac functions by both phasic modifications in reflex mechanisms and by direct descending neural activities. Exactly how certain psychological states such as the one produced by the aversive conditioning paradigm affect the complex cardiovascular dynamics is not clear. It is evident, however, that a higher cerebral system involving the frontal lobe is crucial in orchestrating the complex network of neural regulators of the cardiac response. The close parallel of the SPs and cardiac changes during acquisition is evidence that they involve the same systems. Our finding that the cardiac component of the aversive conditioned response is eliminated by ITP blockade is direct evidence that the MTFCS is, indeed, involved in the regulation of cardiac events in at least this one specific anxiety-evoking situation.

Knowledge of the brain mechanisms involved in the regulation of cardiovascular responses to anxiety-evoking situations is important because a large portion of the sudden deaths (heart attack) unexplained at autopsy [MORITZ and ZAMCHECK, 1946; SPIEKERMAN et al., 1962; KULLER et al., 1966] may be related to episodes of psychological stress. Recently, it has been shown that life changes, such as death of a spouse, recent loss of job, etc., are as significantly correlated with the precipitation of cardiac sudden death as are the physical risk factors high blood pressure and high serum cholesterol [RAHE et al., 1973]. Experiments in our laboratory have shown in an animal model an effect similar to that of life change. Acute coronary occlusion alone was found not to be sufficient to produce ventricular fibrillation and sudden death. Rather an anxiety-related psychological state (e.g. unfamiliarity with the laboratory, periodic electric shock) that was mediated by the nervous system had to accompany the myocardial ischemia in order to initiate the cardiac event of fibrillation [SKINNER et al., 1975a]. Whether or not psychological stress alone can initiate ventricular fibrillation is not known, but direct hypothalamic stimulation can produce arrhythmias [WEINBERG and FUSTER, 1960; MANNING and COTTEN, 1962; MAUCK et al., 1964; GARVEY and MELVILLE, 1969] and eventually, myocardial damage [MELVILLE et al., 1963].

Another line of evidence connecting the MTFCS with the regulation of the myocardium is our recent finding that SWS, characterized by intense electrocortical synchrony, is associated with an increase in ventricular arrhythmias in the infarcted heart [SKINNER et al., 1975b]. Earlier, we showed that ITP lesions eliminate the characteristic 8–12 Hz sleep spindles without affecting other synchronous activities [SKINNER, 1971b]. MUKHAMETOV et al. [1970] and LAMARRE et al. [1971] have shown that R manifests characteristic burst-pause patterns of unit activity only during slow wave episodes in the sleep cycle. These studies indicate that MTFCS and R are, indeed, involved to some extent in SWS processes, but just how the deleterious cardiac events arise during sleep is as yet unknown.

The various types of evoked bioelectric activities discussed above have served as useful probes by which to investigate some of the higher nervous mechanisms that regulate cardiovascular dynamics, mechanisms which have been inaccessible to investigation by other methods. Future analysis of the coupling of frontal SP and aversive conditioned cardiac responses may lend insight into one of the mechanisms mediating the effects of psychological stress on sudden death.

### D. Is the Study of Attention Proper?

The rise and dominance of logical positivism in the psychology of the 1930s under the rubric Behaviorism, forced the shelving of such mentalistic, undefinable yet knowable concepts as 'attention'. At least two significant developments have occurred since then which have tended to bring back into focus the usefulness of certain mentalistic concepts. The first is that logical positivism itself is being successfully attacked by arguments that the observer in the schema is not a passive element. For example, POLANYI [1965] argues that the observer brings tacit knowledge to the situation in order to understand the rational, logical, verbal exposition; i.e. we know more than we can tell. SPERRY's [1974] work on commissurotomy (split-brain) patients indicates that each intact brain contains not only a verbal, analytic, cognitive processor, but a nonverbal, direct-perceptual, synthetic one as well, a finding which constitutes neurophysiological evidence supporting the position that all knowledge is not necessarily obtained by rational or logical verbal processes. Lord RUSSELL said that the ambiguity of axiomatic statements tended to 'unhinge his mind' [GEERTZ, 1965]. What the nonverbal (axiomatic) hemisphere knows simply is not understood by the verbal one, yet the integrated brain uses both cognitive processors together to deal with the world. The second reason for the reinstatement of mentalistic concepts in the behavioral and biological sciences is that biologists never really did abandon the mentalistic practice of functionalism. For example, it has always been acceptable to state that the kidney functions to clean the blood or that the x neural system of the brain functions to produce the x phenomenon, but it is understood that a description of the mechanism must be at hand to support this statement of function. In biology, it is the *pursuit of the physical mechanism* that is the proper scientific activity, and the functional idea helps to formulate the problem pursued.

Our results show that a common system (MTFCS-MRF-R) regulates three types of bioelectric activities (sensory EPs, EEG synchronization, and SP shifts) during certain experimental situations which we consider to be related to the function of attention. Our collective results enable us to support a hypothetical neural model that predicts what our common sense dictates about the mechanism of attention. JAMES [1890] has elegantly articulated what is obvious about attention. The direction of attention is: (1) to external or internal sources; (2) by inherent (innate) or derived (conditioned) features of the stimulus, and (3) either reflexively or voluntarily shifted. The behavioral analysis and electrophysiological features of our model suggest that two systems, the MTFCS and MRF, converge upon an inhibitory gating mechanism, R, which in turn regulates the transmission of information through the sensory relay nuclei of the thalamus. The MTFCS organizes patterns of activity in a topographically organized network that regulates phasic shifts of the bioelectric activities, whereas the MRF maintains a level of activity in a diffusely organized network that tonically regulates the same bioelectric activities. The MTFCS appears to regulate behavior by enabling the animal to inhibit the ascent to the cortex of information evoked by irrelevant stimuli, whereas the MRF appears to regulate more primitive behaviors such as orienting reactions. The conclusion is that the MTFCS regulates the selective and voluntary types of 'attention', whereas the MRF seems to control the more general and reflexive types.

### E. Does our Animal Model Explain Human Attention?

We do not come to know what attention is by observing the behavior of animals or of each other, but by observing our own subjective experiences. Such experiences can be elicited by direct electrical stimulation of the appropriate parts of the brain, and we are thus led to believe that detectable neurophysiological processes underly those phenomenological experiences. A satisfactory experimental approach to attention must attempt to correlate measurements of neurophysiological processes with the subjective experience of attention rather than solely with the objective features of attentive behaviors.

In presenting an animal model of attention, we do not pretend to have dealt in a definitive manner with all of the complexities of the phenomena of attention. We do suggest, however, that our formulation, involving a highly selective gating mechanism operating not at the sensory periphery, but at the thalamocortical levels of information processing, and capable of being overriden by a lower brain stem reflexive mechanism, offers a novel framework for future investigations of mechanisms underlying complex experiential phenomena. For example, the dual control of the thalamic gates by cortical and brain stem mechanisms quite obviously parallels two of the most salient subjective characteristics of attention, the selective filtering of sensory experience and the overriding of volitional attention by reflexive orienting mechanisms.

Our model may be able to explain many of the results concerning event-related potentials in humans, but with the caveat that the frontal SPs and sensory EPs of the cat may not be exactly translatable to the human CNV or the longer latency sensory EPs. Because the MRF and MTFCS can regulate independently the same evoked activity, it is apparent that subtle differences among similar experimental situations may produce strikingly different EP results. For example, a stimulus that is more or less novel may produce very different results in selective discrimination experiments. Each of the three types of evoked bioelectric activity regulated by the MRF and MTFCS seems to reflect different components in the neural processing. Complex interaction between these two systems which regulate the EPs could explain how in various situations the CNV and P300 are sometimes correlated and sometimes independent. The EP features may reflect subtle variations in the two variables related to the MTFCS and MRF, namely the degree of sensory filtering and the amount of reflexive orientation. Recent evidence in humans emphasizes hemispheric laterality of EP components [cf. this series, vol. 3]. Unfortunately, this laterality of hemispheric function does not appear to be manifested in animals. It would seem then that in order to extend our model to the human case, we must posit an extra control on the thalamocortical switching mechanism to channel signals to one hemisphere or the other. It may be that this added control originates in the frontal lobes that part of the mammalian brain which is distinctively human.

## Acknowledgments

This work was supported at various points by Grants HL 05435, HL 13837, and HL 17907 from the National Heart and Lung Institute, NIH, USPHS. C. D. YINGLING was a National Science Foundation Graduate Fellow. The assistance of GREGORY L. KING is greatly appreciated.

## References

ADAMETZ, J. H.: Rate of recovery of functioning in cats with rostral reticular lesions. J. Neurosurg. 16: 85–98 (1959).

ANDERSEN, P. and ECCLES, J. C.: Inhibitory phasing of neuronal discharge. Nature, Lond. 196: 645–647 (1962).

ANDERSEN, P.; ECCLES, J. C., and SEARS, T. A.: The ventro-basal complex of the thalamus: types of cells, their responses and their functional organization. J. Physiol., Lond. 174: 370–399 (1964).

ANDERSEN, P. and SEARS, T. A.: The role of inhibition in the phasing of spontaneous thalamocortical discharge. J. Physiol., Lond. 173: 459–480 (1964).

ARDUINI, A.; MANCIA, M., and MECHELSE, K.: Slow potential changes in the cerebral cortex by sensory and reticular stimulation. Arch. ital. Biol. 95: 127–138 (1957).

BATINI, C.; MAGNI, F.; PALESTINI, M.; ROSSI, G. F., and ZANCHETTI, A.: Neural mechanisms underlying the enduring EEG and behavioral activation in the midpontine pretrigeminal cat. Arch. ital. Biol. 97: 13–25 (1959).

BATSEL, H. L.: Electroencephalographic synchronization and desynchronization in the chronic 'cerveau isolé' of the dog. Electroenceph. clin. Neurophysiol. 12: 421–430 (1960).

BREMER, F. et STOUPEL, N.: Facilitation et inhibition des potentiels évoqués corticaux dans l'éveil cérébral. Archs int. Physiol. Biochim. 67: 240–275 (1959).

BROOKHART, J. M.; ARDUINI, A.; MANCIA, M., and MORUZZI, G.: Thalamocortical relations as revealed by induced slow potential changes. J. Neurophysiol. 21: 499–525 (1958).

BRUTKOWSKI, S.: Prefrontal cortex and drive inhibition; in WARREN and AKERT The frontal granular cortex and behavior, pp. 242–270 (McGraw-Hill, New York 1964).

BUCHWALD, N. A.; WYERS, E. J.; LAUPRECHT, C. W., and HEUSER, G.: The 'caudate spindle'. IV. A behavioral index of caudate-induced inhibition. Electroenceph. clin. Neurophysiol. 13: 531–537 (1961).

BUSER, P.; ROUGEUL, A., and PERRET, C.: Caudate and thalamic influences on conditioned motor responses in the cat. Bol. Inst. Estud. méd. biol. *22:* 293–307 (1964).

CASPERS, H.: Relations of steady potential shifts in the cortex to the wakefulness-sleep spectrum; in BRAZIER Brain function. Cortical excitability and steady potentials, vol. 1, pp. 177–213 (University of California Press, Berkeley 1963).

CASPERS, H.: Shifts of the cortical steady potential during various stages of sleep; in JOUVET Aspects anatomo-fonctionnels de la physiologie du sommeil. Coll. Int. du Centre National de la Recherche Scientifique, No. 127, pp. 213–229, Paris 1965.

CASTELLUCCI, V. F. and GOLDRING, S.: Contribution to steady potential shifts of slow depolarization in cells presumed to be glia. Electroenceph. clin. Neurophysiol. *28:* 109–118 (1970).

CORDEAU, J. P.; WALSH, J. et MAHUT, H.: Variations dans la transmission des messages sensoriels en fonction des différents états d'éveil et de sommeil; in JOUVET Aspects anatomo-fonctionnels de la physiologie du sommeil. Colloques Internationaux du Centre National de la Recherche Scientifique, No. 127, pp. 477–508, Paris 1965.

DAHL, E.; GJERSTAD, L. I., and SKREDE, K. K.: Persistent thalamic and cortical barbiturate spindle activity after ablation of the orbital cortex in cats. Electroenceph. clin. Neurophysiol. *33:* 485–496 (1972).

DEMPSEY, E. W. and MORISON, R. S.: The production of rhythmically recurrent cortical potentials after localized thalamic stimulation. Am. J. Physiol. *135:* 293–300 (1942a).

DEMPSEY, E. W. and MORISON, R. S.: The interaction of certain spontaneous and induced cortical potentials. Am. J. Physiol. *135:* 301–308 (1942b).

DESIRAJU, T. and PURPURA, D. P.: Organization of specific-nonspecific thalamic internuclear synaptic pathways. Brain. Res. *21:* 169–181 (1970).

DOTY, R. W.; BECK, E. C., and KOOI, K. A.: Effect of brain stem lesions on conditioned responses of cats. Expl Neurol. *1:* 360–385 (1959).

DUMONT, S. et DELL, P.: Facilitation réticulaire des mécanismes visuels corticaux. Electroenceph. clin. Neurophysiol. *12:* 769–796 (1960).

EVANS, C. R. and MULHOLLAND, T. B. (eds.): Attention in neurophysiology. Int. Conf. (Appleton Century Crofts, New York 1969).

GARVEY, H. L. and MELVILLE, K. I.: Cardiovascular effects of lateral hypothalamic stimulation in normal and coronary-ligated dogs. J. cardiovasc. Surg. *10:* 377–385 (1969).

GOLDRING, S. and O'LEARY, J. L.: Cortical D.C. changes incident to midline thalamic stimulation. Electroenceph. clin. Neurophysiol. *9:* 577–584 (1957).

GROSSMAN, R. G. and ROSMAN, L. J.: Intracellular potentials of inexcitable cells in epileptogenic cortex undergoing fibrillary gliosis after local injury. Brain Res. *28:* 181–201 (1971).

JAMES, W.: The principles of psychology, vol. 1 (Dover, New York [1890], 1950).

JASPER, H. H.: Diffuse projection systems. The integrative action of the thalamic reticular system. Electroenceph. clin. Neurophysiol. *1:* 405–420 (1949).

JASPER, H. H.: Unspecific thalamocortical relations; in FIELD Handbook of physiology. Neurophysiology, sect. 1, vol. 2, pp. 1307–1321 (Am. Physiological Society, Washington 1960).

JASPER, H. H. and AJMONE-MARSAN, C.: Thalamo-cortical integrating mechanisms. Res. Publ. Ass. nerv. ment. Dis. *30:* 493–512 (1952).

JONES, E. G.: Somes aspects of the organization of the thalamic reticular complex. J. comp. Neurol. *162:* 295–308 (1975).

KONORSKI, J. and LAWICKA, W.: Analysis of errors by prefrontal animals on the delayed-response test; in WARREN and AKERT The frontal granular cortex and behavior, pp. 271–294 (McGraw-Hill, New York 1964).

KULLER, L.; LILIENFELD, A., and FISHER, R.: Epidemiological study of sudden and unexpected deaths to arteriosclerotic heart disease. Circulation *34:* 1056–1068 (1966).

LAMARRE, Y.; FILION, M., and CORDEAU, J. P.: Neuronal discharges of the ventrolateral nucleus of the thalamus during sleep and wakefulness in the cat. I. Spontaneous activity. Expl Brain Res. *12:* 480–498 (1971).

LINDSLEY, D. B.: Attention, consciousness, sleep and wakefulness; in FIELD Handbook of Physiology. Neurophysiology, sect. 1, vol. 3, pp. 1553–1593 (Am. Physiological Society, Washington 1960).

LINDSLEY, D. B.; SCHREINER, L. H.; KNOWLES, W. B., and MAGOUN, H. W.: Behavioral and EEG changes following chronic brain stem lesions in the cat. Electroenceph. clin. Neurophysiol. *2:* 483–498 (1950).

LOTHMAN, E.; LAMANNA, J.; CORDINGLEY, G.; ROSENTHAL, M., and SOMJEN, G. G.: Responses of electrical potentials, potassium levels and oxidative metabolic activity of the cerebral neocortex of cats. Brain Res. *88:* 15–36 (1975).

LOTHMAN, E. W. and SOMJEN, G. G.: Extracellular potassium activity, intracellular and extracellular potential responses in the spinal cord. J. Physiol., Lond. *252:* 115–136 (1975).

LURIA, A. R. and HOMSKAYA, E. D.: Frontal lobes and the regulation of arousal processes; in MOSTOFSKY Attention: contemporary theory and analysis, pp. 303–330 (Appleton Century Crofts, New York 1970).

MAGOUN, H. W.: The waking brain, p. 174 (Thomas, Springfield 1963).

MAHUT, H.: Effects of subcortical electrical stimulation on discrimination learning in cats. J. comp. physiol. Psychol. *58:* 390–395 (1964).

MANNING, J. W. and COTTEN, M. DE V.: Mechanism of cardiac arrhythmias induced by diencephalic stimulation. Am. J. Physiol. *203:* 1120–1124 (1962).

MARK, R. G. and HALL, R. D.: Acoustically evoked potentials in the rat during conditioning. J. Neurophysiol. *30:* 875–892 (1967).

MAUCK, H. P.; HOCKMAN, C. H., and HOFF, E. C.: ECG changes after cerebral stimulation. I. Anomalous atrioventricular excitation elicited by electrical stimulation of the mesencephalic reticular formation. Am. Heart J. *68:* 98–101 (1964).

MELVILLE, K. I.; BLUM, B.; SHISTER, H. E., and SILVER, M. D.: Cardiac ischemic changes and arrhythmias induced by hypothalamic stimulation. Am J. Cardiol. *12:* 781–791 (1963).

MILLHOUSE, O. E.: A Golgi study of the descending medial forebrain bundle. Brain Res. *15:* 341–363 (1969).

MISHKIN, M.: Perseveration of central sets after frontal lesions in monkeys; in WAR-

REN and AKERT The frontal granular cortex and behavior, pp. 219–241 (McGraw-Hill, New York 1964).

MORISON, R. S. and DEMPSEY, E. W.: A study of thalamocortical relations. Am. J. Physiol. *135:* 281–292 (1942).

MORISON, R. S. and DEMPSEY. E. W.: Mechanism of thalamocortical augmentation and repetition. Am. J. Physiol. *138:* 297–308 (1943).

MORITZ, A. R. and ZAMCHECK, N.: Sudden and unexpected death of young soldiers. Archs Path. *42:* 459–494 (1946).

MORUZZI, G. and MAGOUN, H. W.: Brain stem reticular formation and activation of the EEG. Electroenceph. clin. Neurophysiol. *1:* 455–473 (1949).

MOSTOFSKY, D. I. (ed.): Attention: contemporary theory and analysis (Appleton Century Crofts, New York 1970).

MUKHAMETOV, L. M.; RIZZOLATTI, G., and TRADARDI, V.: Spontaneous activity of neurons of nucleus reticularis thalami in freely moving cats. J. Physiol., Lond. *210:* 651–667 (1970).

NAUTA, W. J. H.: Some efferent connections of the prefrontal cortex in the monkey; in WARREN and AKERT The frontal granular cortex and behavior, pp. 397–409 (McGraw-Hill, New York 1964).

PECCI-SAVAADRA, J.; DOTY, R. W., and HUNT, H. B.: Conditioned reflexes elicited in squirrel monkeys by stimuli producing recruiting responses. Electroenceph. clin. Neurophysiol. *19:* 492–500 (1965).

POLANYI, M.: The structure of consciousness. Brain *88:* 799–810 (1965).

PURPURA, D. P. and COHEN, B.: Intracellular recording from thalamic neurons during recruiting responses. J. Neurophysiol. *25:* 621–635 (1962).

PURPURA, D. P.; FRIGYESI, T. L.; MCMURTRY, J. G., and SCARFF, T.: Synaptic mechanisms in thalamic regulation of cerebello-cortical projection activity; in PURPURA and YAHR The thalamus, pp. 153–172 (Columbia University Press, New York 1966).

RAHE, R. H.; BENNETT, L.; ROMO, M.; SILTANEN, P., and ARTHUR, R. J.: Subjects' recent life changes and coronary heart disease in Finland. Am. J. Psychiat. *130:* 1222–1226 (1973).

RAMÓN Y CAJAL, S.: Histologie du système nerveux de l'homme et des vertébrés, vol. 2 (Maloine, Paris 1911).

ROBERTSON, R. T. and LYNCH, G. S.: Orbitofrontal modulation of EEG spindles. Brain Res. *28:* 562–566 (1971).

ROSE, J.: The cortical connections of the reticular complex of the thalamus. Res. Publ. Ass. nerv. ment. Dis. *30:* 454–479 (1952).

ROSSI, G. F.; PALESTINI, M.; PISANO, M., and ROSADINI, G.: An experimental study of the cortical reactivity during sleep and wakefulness; in JOUVET Aspects anatomo-fonctionnels de la physiologie du sommeil. Coll. Int. du Centre National de la Recherche Scientifique, No. 127, pp. 509–532, Paris 1965.

SCHEIBEL, M. E. and SCHEIBEL, A. B.: The organization of the nucleus reticularis thalami: a Golgi study. Brain Res. *1:* 43–62 (1966).

SCHEIBEL, M. E. and SCHEIBEL, A. B.: Structural organization of nonspecific thalamic nuclei and their projection toward cortex. Brain Res. *6:* 60–94 (1967).

SCHEIBEL, M. E. and SCHEIBEL, A. B.: Specialized organizational patterns within the nucleus reticularis thalami of the cat. Expl Neurol. *34:* 316–322 (1972).

SCHLAG, J. and VILLABLANCA, J.: Cortical incremental responses to thalamic stimulation. Brain Res. *6:* 119–142 (1967).

SCHLAG, J. and WASZAK, M.: Characteristics of unit responses in nucleus reticularis thalami. Brain Res. *21:* 286–288 (1970).

SCHLAG, J. D. and WASZAK, M.: Electrophysiological properties of units of the thalamic reticular complex. Expl Neurol. *32:* 79–97 (1971).

SKINNER, J. E.: Electrocortical desynchronization during functional blockade of the mesencephalic reticular formation. Brain Res. *22:* 254–258 (1970a).

SKINNER, J. E.: Neuroscience: a laboratory manual (Saunders, Philadelphia 1971a).

SKINNER, J. E.: A cryoprobe and cryoplate for reversible functional blockade in the brains of chronic animal preparations. Electroenceph. clin. Neurophysiol. *29:* 204–205 (1970b).

SKINNER, J. E.: Abolition of several forms of cortical synchronization during blockade in the inferior thalamic peduncle. Electroenceph. clin. Neurophysiol. *31:* 211–221 (1971b).

SKINNER, J. E.: Abolition of a conditioned, surface-negative, cortical potential during cryogenic blockade of the non-specific thalamocortical system. Electroenceph. clin. Neurophysiol. *31:* 197–209 (1971c).

SKINNER, J. E.; LIE, J. T., and ENTMAN, M. L.: Modification of ventricular fibrillation latency following coronary artery occlusion in the conscious pig. The effects of psychological stress and beta-adrenergic blockade. Circulation *51:* 656–667 (1975a).

SKINNER, J. E. and LINDSLEY, D. B.: Electrophysiological and behavioral effects of blockade of the nonspecific thalamo-cortical system. Brain Res. *6:* 95–118 (1967).

SKINNER, J. E. and LINDSLEY, D. B.: Reversible cryogenic blockade of neural function in the brain of unrestrained animals. Science *161:* 595–597 (1968).

SKINNER, J. E. and LINDSLEY, D. B.: Enhancement of visual and auditory evoked potentials during blockade of the nonspecific thalamo-cortical system. Electroenceph. clin. Neurophysiol. *31:* 1–6 (1971).

SKINNER, J. E.; MOHR, D. N., and KELLAWAY, P.: Modification of arrhythmia rate and ventricular fibrillation latency following coronary occlusion in the unanesthetized pig. Effects of the stages of sleep. Circulation Res. *37:* 342–349 (1975b).

SKINNER, J. E. and YINGLING, C. D.: Regulation of slow potential shifts in nucleus reticularis thalami by the mesencephalic reticular formation and the frontal granular cortex. Electroenceph. clin. Neurophysiol. *40:* 288–296 (1976).

SMITH, O. A.: Reflex and central mechanisms involved in the control of the heart and ciuculation. Ann. Rev. Physiol. *36:* 93–123 (1974).

SMITH, O. A.; NATHAN, M. A., and CLARKE, N. P.: Central nervous system pathways mediating blood pressure changes; in WOOD Hypertension. Neural control of arterial pressure, vol. 16, pp. 9–22 (Am. Heart Association, New York 1968).

SPERRY, R. W.: Lateral specialization in the surgically separated hemispheres; in SCHMITT and WORDEN The neurosciences. 3rd Study Program, pp. 5–19 (MIT Press, Cambridge 1974).

SPIEKERMAN, R. E.; BRANDENBURG, J. T.; ACHOR, R. W. P., and EDWARDS, J. E.: The spectrum of coronary heart disease in a community of 30,000. Circulation 25: 57–65 (1962).

SPRAGUE, J. M.; CHAMBERS, W. W., and STELLAR, E.: Attentive, affective and adaptive behavior in the cat. Science 133: 165–173 (1961).

STAUNTON, H. P. and SASAKI, K.: Recruiting responses not dependent on orbitofrontal cortex. Brain Res. 30: 415–418 (1971).

VELASCO, M. and LINDSLEY, D. B.: Role of orbital cortex in regulation of thalamo-cortical electrical activity. Science 149: 1375–1377 (1965).

VELASCO, M.; SKINNER, J. E.; ASARO, K. D., and LINDSLEY, D. B.: Thalamo-cortical systems regulating spindle bursts and recruiting responses. I. Effect of cortical ablations. Electroenceph. clin. Neurophysiol. 25: 463–470 (1968).

VILLABLANCA, J.: The electrocorticogram in the chronic cerveau isolé cat. Electroenceph. clin. Neurophysiol. 19: 576–586 (1965).

WASZAK, M.: Effect of polarizing currents on potentials evoked in neurons of the ventral leaf of nucleus reticularis thalami by intralaminar stimulation. Expl Neurol. 40: 82–89 (1973).

WASZAK, M.: Effect of barbiturate anesthesia on discharge pattern in nucleus reticularis thalami. Pharmac. biochem. Behav. 2: 339–345 (1974).

WEINBERG, S. J. and FUSTER, J. M.: Electrocardiographic changes produced by localized hypothalamic stimulations. Ann. intern. Med. 53: 332–341 (1960).

Prof. JAMES E. SKINNER, Neurophysiology Section, Physiology Department, Baylor College of Medicine, Houston, TX 77030 (USA). Tel. (713) 790 3105.

Dr. CHARLES D. YINGLING, Langley Porter Neuropsychiatric Institute, University of California, 401 Parnassus Avenue, San Francisco, CA 94143 (USA). Tel. (415) 681 8080.

Attention, Voluntary Contraction and Event-Related Cerebral Potentials.
Prog. clin. Neurophysiol., vol. 1, Ed. J. E. Desmedt, pp. 70–96 (Karger, Basel 1977)

# Gating of Thalamic Input to Cerebral Cortex by Nucleus Reticularis Thalami

Charles D. Yingling and James E. Skinner

Neurophysiology Section, Physiology Department, Baylor College of Medicine, Houston, Tex.

Nucleus reticularis thalami (R) is a thin sheet of cells of ventral thalamic origin that surrounds the thalamus. Its anterior pole has major interconnections with both the mesencephalic reticular formation (MRF) and the mediothalamic-frontocortical system (MTFCS) [Scheibel and Scheibel, 1966]. All thalamocortical and corticothalamic fibers from both specific and nonspecific systems must pass through R on their way to and from the cerebral cortex. R was once considered as the final common pathway for nonspecific thalamic projections onto cortex [Jasper, 1949; Rose and Woolsey, 1949], but Golgi studies and axonal transport have now shown that nearly all R axons project back into the thalamus rather than radially toward the cortex [Ramón y Cajal, 1909–1911; Scheibel and Scheibel, 1966; Jones, 1975]. Anatomical studies which suggested the possibility of R-cortical pathways [Rose and Woolsey, 1949; Chow, 1952; Rose, 1952; Carman et al., 1964] can be more satisfactorily explained by considering the degeneration found in R after cortical lesions to be transneuronal in origin. Thus, unless new anatomical evidence is found to suggest the presence of cortical projections of R, it would seem to be more prudent to assume an exclusively thalamic destination for axons leaving the confines of R. R seems to be in a unique strategic position to influence virtually all thalamic and cortical activities in either a generalized or a selective manner. Recent physiological studies have shown striking inverse correlations between firing patterns of cells in R and adjoining areas of nucleus ventralis lateralis (VL) [Schlag and Waszak, 1970, 1971; Filion et al., 1971; Frigyesi, 1971, 1972; Frigyesi and

SCHWARTZ, 1972], a finding that suggests that R may exert an inhibitory effect on thalamic nuclei. The possibility that R may function as a topographically specific inhibitory feedback circuit makes it a prime candidate for selective regulation of thalamocortical activities. The results reported here indeed suggest that: (1) R is capable of selectively gating transmission through major thalamic relay nuclei, thus controlling the amplitude of cortical EPs; (2) unit activities in R are correlated with the production of IPSPs in the thalamus associated with 8- to 12-Hz synchronous activity, and (3) large slow-potential (SP) shifts in R, reflecting major changes in patterns of unit activity, accompany behavioral states of arousal, orienting, expectancy, and selective perception. This manuscript contains new results and also reviews a series of three recent papers from our laboratory [YINGLING and SKINNER, 1975, 1976; SKINNER and YINGLING, 1976]. Together, these results provide a current view on the gating of thalamic input to cerebral cortex by R.

## Methods

A total of 30 adult cats was used. With the exception of the unit recordings, all major results obtained in acute unanesthetized preparations have been replicated in at least three unrestrained chronic preparations. Bipolar stainless steel stimulating electrodes, platinized-platinum recording electrodes, tungsten microelectrodes, and cryoprobes for temporary functional blockade [SKINNER, 1971a] were stereotaxically implanted under ether or short-acting barbiturate (pentothal) anesthesia. Acute preparations were then infiltrated with Lidocaine at all wound edges, immobilized with Flaxedil (gallamine triethiodide), and artificially ventilated through an endotracheal tube. Normal body temperature was maintained with a heating pad. Recordings were not begun for 2–4 h after the effects of the anesthesia had worn off, as determined by the return of spontaneous and evoked cortical activity to a normal appearance. The ventilation was adjusted to maintain the animal in an optimally responsive state, as determined by the following criteria: (1) desynchronized EEG; (2) resting pupil diameter of approximately 2–3 mm under normal room illumination; (3) pupillary dilation in response to stroking or manipulation of joints, which proved to be the best single test of responsiveness. Blood samples were periodically analyzed on a Corning 165 blood-gas analyzer as a check for maintenance of $pO_2$, $pCO_2$, and pH within normal levels. A rigorous control was thus maintained over the state of ventilation to avoid any slight deviations from the normal acid-base balance which would modify slow potential shifts.

At the conclusion of an acute experiment, the effect of Flaxedil was allowed to wear off, and within 1–2 h, the animal would be sitting up and breathing regularly, appearing normally alert. This rapid recovery served as a further check and had the further advantage of allowing an animal with fortuitous electrode placements to be converted into a chronic preparation for behavioral studies. Chronic animals were prepared by securing all leads in a protective cap of dental acrylic and allowing the animals to recover from surgery until they were eating and drinking normally.

Electrical stimuli were delivered by Grass S-8 stimulators, via stimulus-isolation units. DC recordings of SPs were referenced to inactive electrodes embedded in Gelfoam, moistened with saline, and placed in the most anterior part of the frontal sinus septal bone. Possible contamination from eye movement potentials were negligible in amplitude and showed no temporal congruence with the evoked SPs. The SPs were recorded on a Beckman Type R polygraph and were sometimes averaged on a CAT 400 computer. Evoked potentials (EPs) were viewed on a Tektronix 555 oscilloscope and recorded on film. Conditioning trials, controlled by BRS solid-state programming apparatus, consisted of a 0.5-sec tone, followed in 4 sec by a mildly noxious shock to the hind limbs (100-Hz, 0.5-msec duration, 30- to 50-msec train) that was delivered through stainless steel wires sutured into the skin.

At the conclusion of the experiments, all animals were anesthetized and perfused through the carotid artery with 40% formaldehyde; the brains were then sectioned at 100 $\mu$m on a freezing microtome. The relevant sections were stained with thionine for histological determination of all electrode and cryoprobe locations [SKINNER, 1971a].

## Results

### A. Terminology

Rather than using descriptive anatomical terminology, we designate areas of R by adding a subscript that denotes the adjoining thalamic nucleus: hence, $R_{VA}$ refers to the anterior pole of R that adjoins nucleus ventralis anterior, $R_{LG}$ lies dorsolateral to the lateral geniculate body, etc. This terminology is simple and identifies that thalamic region with which a given segment of R is most likely to have functional relationships.

### B. Reduction of EPs by Stimulation of Various Regions of Nucleus Reticularis Thalami

Visual evoked potentials (VEPs) to stimulation of the optic tract (OT) were recorded over ipsilateral primary visual cortex. Prior to the OT stimulus, a 30 msec train of pulses at 250 Hz was delivered through a second stimulating electrode in $R_{LG}$. All components of the VEP were abolished or highly attenuated by $R_{LG}$ stimulation at any time within the 100 msec prior to OT stimulation; the effect was absent or much weaker when stimulating on either side of $R_{LG}$, i.e. in optic radiations (OR) or lateral geniculate nucleus (LGN). This control excludes the possibility of the effect being due to cortical recovery cycles. This control was necessary,

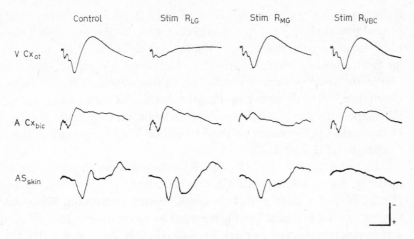

Fig. 1. Inhibition of EPs in three major sense modalities by stimulation of R. In this and all subsequent figures, unless otherwise noted, capital letters refer to recording sites; lower case letters refer to stimulation sites. Subscripts $R_{LG}$, etc., refer to the thalamic nucleus adjoining the area of R being studied. VEPs were elicited by optic tract (ot) stimulation and recorded in primary visual cortex (V Cx); AEPs were elicited by stimulation of the brachium of the inferior colliculus (bic) and recorded in primary auditory cortex (A Cx); SEPs were elicited by stimulation of stainless steel wires sutured through the skin and recorded in sensorimotor cortex (lateral AS). 50 msec prior to the evoking stimulus, a train of 20 msec at 250 Hz was delivered to either $R_{LG}$, $R_{MG}$, or $R_{VBC}$. $R_{LG}$ stimulation attenuates the VEP but has no effect on the AEP or SEP; similarly, $R_{MG}$ stimulation affects only the AEP and stimulation of $R_{VBC}$ affects only the SEP. In each case, both early and late components of the EP are affected. Calibration: 200 $\mu$V; 4 msec (VEPs), 10 msec (AEPs, SEPs). From YINGLING and SKINNER [1976].

since any stimulus to $R_{LG}$ inevitably excited the thalamocortical fibers of passage as well, thus giving rise to a cortical EP. However, stimulation within LG or OR adjacent to $R_{LG}$ also stimulated these thalamocortical fibers and produced cortical EPs; since these conditioning stimuli did not have the same effect on OT-evoked test EPs, the effects observed must be due to a specific inhibitory effect of cells in $R_{LG}$. Stimulation of $R_{MG}$ or $R_{VBC}$ had no effect on OT-evoked VEPs, and stimulation of $R_{LG}$ had no effect on nonprimary EPs to OT stimuli recorded in auditory cortex. Unilateral $R_{LG}$ stimulation was effective in reducing VEPs to *photic* stimuli only if the stimulus was localized in the visual half field opposite to the site of $R_{LG}$ stimulation, which indicates that the effect was ipsilateral.

Due to the bilateral representation of auditory information in the thalamus, $R_{MG}$ stimulation on one side was ineffective in reducing auditory evoked potentials (AEPs) to binaural click stimuli. However, when electrically stimulating the brachium of the inferior colliculus (BIC) just posterior to the medial geniculate (MGB), a condition analogous to OT stimulation in the visual system, a parallel result was obtained: $R_{MG}$ stimulation during the 100 msec preceding the stimulus to BIC reduced or abolished all components of the AEP. Again, stimulation on either side of $R_{MG}$, i.e. in the auditory radiations or the MGB, had little or no effect, nor did stimulation of $R_{LG}$ or $R_{VBC}$.

In order to test the effect of R stimulation on the somatosensory modality, $R_{VBC}$, which projects axons back into the ventrobasal complex (VBC), was stimulated prior to a shock applied to the skin. The somatosensory evoked potential (SEP), recorded in anterior sigmoid (AS) cortex, was completely blocked by prior $R_{VBC}$ stimulation, but was not affected by $R_{MG}$ or $R_{LG}$ stimuli.

These results are summarized in figure 1, which documents the topographical specificity of the inhibitory effect [YINGLING and SKINNER, 1976].

### C. Unit Responses in Nucleus Reticularis Thalami during Recruiting Responses and Reticular Activation

Intracellular recordings in the thalamus during recruiting responses (RR) have demonstrated prolonged IPSPs in VL following medial thalamic stimulation, inhibitory events which appear to underlie the timing of the basic 8- to 12-Hz frequency of spontaneous or induced spindle activity [PURPURA and COHEN, 1962]. During these IPSPs, monosynaptic transmission through VL is effectively blocked [PURPURA et al., 1965, 1966a]. The following experiments were performed to test a hypothesis [SCHEIBEL and SCHEIBEL, 1967] that activities originating in R could be related to the generation of these IPSPs.

Recruiting responses (RRs) elicited by 8-Hz stimulation of nucleus centralis medialis (NCM), and recorded in AS cortex, were displayed on the first beam of the oscilloscope, while unit activity in $R_{VA}$ and $R_{VL}$ was displayed on the second beam. Units that were later found to be in the VA or VL nuclei of the thalamus responded to each stimulus with a brief burst of one to a few spikes at a latency of 8–10 msec (fig. 2). The interneuronal pathway mediating this fairly long latency of activation is unknown [PURPURA, 1970]. Units encountered at the anterior borders of the thalamus, which proved to be in $R_{VA}$ or occasionally in medial parts of

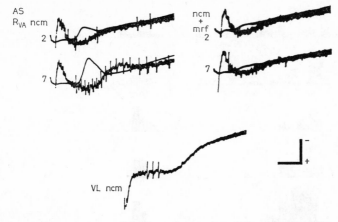

*Fig. 2.* Unit activity in nucleus reticularis thalami ($R_{VA}$) and VL during RRs. Upper traces show a unit in $R_{VA}$ together with the cortical response recorded in medial AS cortex; the lower centered trace shows a unit in VL. Top left, responses to the second and seventh stimuli in a train (1 sec, 8 Hz) delivered to nucleus centralis medialis (ncm); note that the recruitment in the cortex is paralleled by an increase in the $R_{VA}$ unit responses from a few spikes to a sustained high-frequency burst, with a latency slightly shorter than the cortical response. Top right, responses when each stimulus to ncm was preceded by a 20-msec, 250-Hz train to the mesencephalic reticular formation (mrf). The cortical response is blocked, as is the unit response in $R_{VA}$. Note also the disappearance of the thalamic RR, which can be seen in the unit trace 7 on the left as a downward (positive) deflection of the baseline at the time of the cortical response. The lower centered trace shows a VL unit responding to the same 8 Hz ncm stimulation with a brief burst of three spikes followed by a prolonged silent period during the high-frequency burst in $R_{VA}$. Calibration: 200 $\mu$V (AS), 50 $\mu$V ($R_{VA}$, VL); 20 msec.

$R_{VL}$, responded with prolonged high-frequency bursts that often extended throughout the interstimulus interval (fig. 2). The latency of these bursts was 10–30 msec (average 20 msec), slightly shorter than the latency of the cortical RRs as well as the thalamic IPSPs previously reported. The burst pattern in $R_{VA}$ cells exhibited a parallel recruitment with the cortical RRs, firing only a few spikes to the first stimulus in each train, but developing sustained bursts at frequencies up to 250–400 Hz by the time of maximal amplitude of the cortical RRs. Modulation of the stimulus amplitude during an extended train produced parallel effects on $R_{VA}$ units and cortical RRs. Stimuli below the threshold for production of cortical responses had no effect on $R_{VA}$ units.

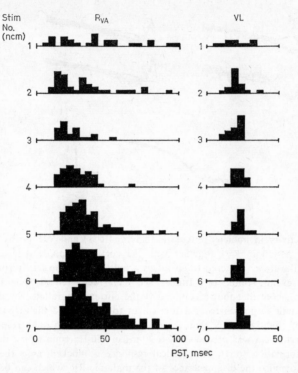

*Fig. 3.* Post-stimulus time (PST) histograms of unit activity evoked in $R_{VA}$ and VL by each of 7 stimuli delivered at 8 Hz to the nucleus centralis medialis (ncm). Pooled results of 12 separate trials. The $R_{VA}$ histograms resemble the IPSPs recorded in VL cells during recruiting responses. The IPSPs and $R_{VA}$ histograms have similar latencies, waveforms, and durations and each shows amplitude recruitment. The VL histograms show a sharp cutoff at the time of the peak of the $R_{VA}$ histograms. Bin width of each histogram is 4.35 msec.

The recruiting character of the responses can be seen most clearly in the post-stimulus time (PST) histograms (fig. 3), for each stimulus in the 8-Hz train averaged over several successive trains. Also noteworthy is the striking resemblance of the histogram envelopes of the $R_{VA}$ responses to the waveforms of IPSPs recorded intracellularly in VL cells during RRs [PURPURA and COHEN, 1962], a finding which suggests a causal relationship between the bursts in $R_{VA}$ and the IPSPs in VL. This suggestion is further supported by the sharp cutoff of the bursts elicited in the VL unit; the VL unit is totally silenced by the time of maximal development of the burst in $R_{VA}$.

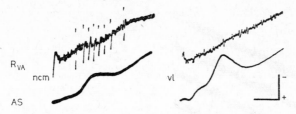

*Fig. 4.* Unit responses in nucleus reticularis thalami ($R_{VA}$) during RRs and ARs. On the left is shown the characteristic high-frequency burst of an $R_{VA}$ unit to one of the later stimuli in a 1-sec, 8-Hz train delivered to nucleus centralis medialis (ncm); the lower trace shows the monophasic negative RR recorded in medial AS cortex. On the right is shown the response of the same $R_{VA}$ unit to stimulation of VL; note the absence of any activation of the unit by this stimulus. The biphasic positive-negative waveform of the augmenting response in AS is seen in the lower trace. Calibration: 50 $\mu$V ($R_{VA}$), 200 $\mu$V (AS); 20 msec.

Stimulation of VL to produce augmenting responses (ARs) was without effect on $R_{VA}$ units that responded vigorously to NCM stimulation (fig. 4). This finding suggests that the medial thalamic IPSPs associated with ARs [DESIRAJU and PURPURA, 1970] are mediated by a separate intrathalamic pathway not involving R.

A 250-msec stimulation of the mesencephalic reticular formation (MRF) at 100 Hz, which desynchronized the spontaneous EEG and reduced the amplitude of RRs, strongly inhibited the spontaneous firing of $R_{VA}$ units, many of which fell completely silent for several seconds (fig. 5) [YINGLING and SKINNER, 1975]. High-frequency stimulation of NCM initially elicited high-frequency firing of $R_{VA}$ units. However, this response lasted only as long as the stimulus train, and was followed by a prolonged depression of firing similar to that produced by MRF stimulation. When low-frequency stimulation of NCM was paired with high-frequency stimulation of MRF, a manipulation that abolished thalamic IPSPs [PURPURA et al., 1966b] as well as thalamic and cortical RRs, the bursting response of $R_{VA}$ units to NCM stimulation was abolished (fig. 2, upper right traces); this finding suggests that the desynchronizing effects of MRF activation may result from inhibition of R cells involved in the production of the IPSPs thought to underlie the thalamo-cortical synchronization.

Cryogenic blockade of the inferior thalamic peduncle (ITP) interconnecting the medial thalamus (MT) and the frontal cortex (FC) abolished cortical *and thalamic* recruiting responses, but not augmenting responses

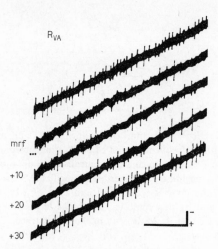

*Fig. 5.* Inhibition of nucleus reticularis thalami ($R_{VA}$) unit responses by mrf stimulation. The top trace shows the spontaneous activity of a unit recorded in $R_{VA}$, firing at an average rate of approximately 40 Hz. A 250-msec, 250-Hz train was delivered to the MRF just prior to the second trace (dots), and immediately the unit is almost totally silenced. The next three traces show samples of the unit's activity recorded 10, 20, and 30 sec after the MRF stimulation. Note the extremely slow recovery of the firing rate, which is still slightly depressed (30 Hz) 30 sec after termination of the stimulus to the MRF. Calibration: 50 $\mu$V; 250 msec. From YINGLING and SKINNER [1975].

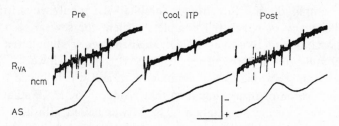

*Fig. 6.* Abolition of unit responses in nucleus reticularis thalami ($R_{VA}$) during cryogenic blockade of the ITP. On the left (Pre) is shown the characteristic high-frequency burst of $R_{VA}$ unit activity in response to medial thalamic (ncm) stimulation; the RR in medial AS cortex is seen in the lower trace. In the Cool ITP condition, the evoked burst of unit activity is abolished together with the cortical response during cooling to 5 °C of bilateral cryoprobes which had been implanted previously in the ITP (Horsley-Clarke coordinates A 13.5, L 3.0, H –3.5). Note that the unit is not inactivated by spread of the cooling gradient into the recording area, as spontaneous spikes are still seen during the blockade. The Post record shows the restoration of both cortical and unit responses 3 min after cessation of cooling. Calibration: 200 $\mu$V (AS), 50 $\mu$V ($R_{VA}$); 20 msec.

[SKINNER and LINDSLEY, 1967]. ITP blockade also was found to abolish the burst responses of $R_{VA}$ units to NCM stimulation (fig. 6). This effect was not due to inactivation of the units by a spread of cooling into the recording area, as the cells still fired occasional spontaneous spikes during the blockade. RRs and $R_{VA}$ burst-responses exhibited a *parallel* return to their normal patterns during rewarming of the tissues. This result suggests that the mechanism involved in the production of the $R_{VA}$ bursts is not entirely dependent on intrathalamic synaptic pathways, but also involves participation of the frontal cortex via the ITP.

In conclusion, the data presented here are consistent with the suggestion that inhibitory projections from cells in $R_{VA}$, activated via a thalamo-cortico-R pathway, are responsible for the prolonged IPSPs observed in thalamic sites during RRs. Desynchronization following MRF activation results from inhibition of R units, thus preventing the generation of synchronizing IPSPs [YINGLING and SKINNER, 1975].

### D. Slow-Potential Shifts in Nucleus Reticularis Thalami Related to Arousal, Orienting, and Expectancy

*1. SPs evoked by MRF stimulation.* Brief high-frequency stimulation of the MRF evoked slow surface-negative shifts in frontal (AS) cortex (transcortical potentials 200–1000 $\mu V$) together with larger positive shifts in $R_{VA}$ or $R_{VL}$ (monopolar potentials 5–10 mV) (fig. 7) [SKINNER and YINGLING, 1976]. Since MRF stimulation produces prolonged inhibition of units in $R_{VA}$ and $R_{VL}$ (fig. 5) [SCHLAG and WASZAK, 1971; WASZAK, 1974], it is likely that this extracellular positivity in R reflects synchronous hyperpolarizations of cells in the vicinity of the recording electrode. Both AS and $R_{VA}$ potentials had identical time courses that peaked slowly at 10–15 sec and required up to 30 sec or more to return to baseline. Occasional large SPs were recorded in $R_{LG}$ following MRF stimulation, but these were much more variable in waveform, amplitude, and time course than potentials recorded in $R_{VA}$ or $R_{VL}$ (fig. 7) [SKINNER and YINGLING, 1976]. Some animals did not show large responses in $R_{LG}$. Such between-animal variabilities may have been due to an inability to place the recording electrode entirely within the very thin segments of R posterior to the neuropil region in $R_{VA}$. These potentials were resistant to habituation, showing no decrement after 200 repetitions at 1 per 30 sec. In chronic preparations, the return to baseline coincided with the cessation of behavioral signs of arousal and orienting following the stimulus. Each stimulus caused an initial jerk and usually a loud vocalization, fol-

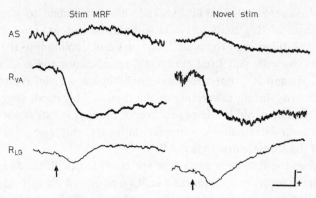

*Fig.* 7. SP responses in FC (medial AS) and nucleus reticularis thalami ($R_{VA}$, $R_{LG}$) accompanying mesencephalic reticular formation stimulation (Stim MRF) and orienting responses (Novel stim). DC coupled recordings are shown from FC (AS) transcortically, and from areas of R adjacent to nucleus ventralis anterior ($R_{VA}$) and the lateral geniculate ($R_{LG}$), both referenced to frontal sinus bone. On the left are shown the responses to 250-msec, 250-Hz stimulation of the MRF (arrow); a surface negative shift of about 1,000 $\mu$V in AS is paralleled by a large (4-mV) positive shift in $R_{VA}$ and a smaller, initially positive shift in $R_{LG}$. On the right, quite similar responses are evoked by a novel stimulus, in this case striking the door of the recording chamber. Calibration: 1,000 $\mu$V; 10 sec. From SKINNER and YINGLING [1975].

lowed by a period in which the animal looked around repeatedly usually in a direction contralateral to the side of the stimulus. As the SPs began to wane, the animal calmed down, and when the SPs approached the baseline, the animal returned to a quiet, resting posture.

The SPs in the cortex were localized in AS and orbitofrontal regions; no SPs were seen in posterior sigmoid, coronal, anterior middle suprasylvian, auditory, or visual cortices. The large subcortical responses were seen only in R. SPs were not seen in recordings from specific relay, association, or medial nonspecific thalamic nuclei. Moving the recording electrode in R by as little as 0.5 mm into the internal capsule resulted in the almost total disappearance of a 12 mV response (fig. 8), which returned when the electrode was again moved back into R [SKINNER and YINGLING, 1976]. Light barbiturate anesthesia resulted in abolition of behavioral and SP responses to MRF stimulation. SP responses returned in parallel with behavioral signs of arousal as the effects of the drug wore off.

High frequency MT stimulation drives $R_{VA}$ units following each stimulus pulse of the train [SCHLAG and WASZAK, 1971]. However, after the

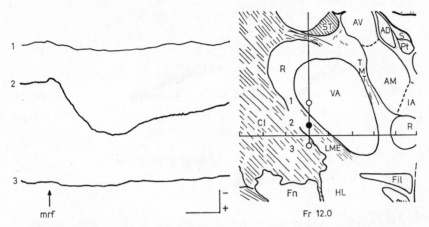

*Fig. 8.* Localization of the SP response in nucleus reticularis thalami ($R_{VA}$) following mesencephalic reticular formation (MRF) stimulation. Three responses to 250-msec, 250-Hz stimulation of the MRF, recorded at the points indicated on the electrode track on the right, are shown. Points 1 and 3, in nucleus ventralis anterior (VA) and the internal capsule (CI), respectively, show little or no response; point 2, in $R_{VA}$, shows a slow positive shift of 12 mV. The three points are each separated by a distance of 1 mm; the recording electrode was moved back and forth between points 2 and 3 several times, and in each case the response was only seen at point 2, in $R_{VA}$. Calibration: 5,000 $\mu$V; 10 sec. From SKINNER and YINGLING [1976].

termination of the train, the phasic activation was followed by a prolonged depression of firing (see section C above) [SCHLAG and WASZAK, 1971], an inhibitory effect which was accompanied by a positive SP in $R_{VA}$ (fig. 9) and a surface-negative SP in FC. The positive SP in $R_{VA}$ is thus once again seen to be associated with inhibition of unit activity, as it was following MRF stimulation. The inhibition in R produced by high frequency MT stimulation may be due to indirect activation of the MRF [SCHLAG and CHAILLET, 1963]. In further support of the MT-MRF-R pathway is our finding that SPs of similar amplitude, wave shape, and time course, were evoked by high-frequency stimulation of either MT or the MRF (fig. 9, control). Furthermore, a negative SP in the MRF is seen during the SPs recorded in FC and $R_{VA}$ following high frequency MT stimulation (fig. 10A).

Functional blockade of the ITP produced sustained surface-negative SPs in FC and positive SPs in $R_{VA}$ (fig. 11). The positive SP in $R_{VA}$ could be due to removal of a tonic depolarizing influence on $R_{VA}$ by the FC. Removal of this steady cortical excitation would result in hyperpolarization

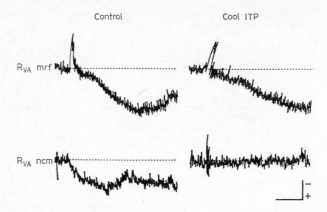

*Fig. 9.* SPs evoked in nucleus reticularis thalami ($R_{VA}$) by MRF and high-frequency medial thalamic (nucleus centralis medialis, ncm) stimulation before (Control) and during (Cool ITP) blockade of the ITP. Control traces show similar positive SPs evoked in $R_{VA}$ by 250-msec, 250-Hz stimulation of either the MRF or MT (ncm). On the right, cooling of the ITP to 5 °C does not affect the response to MRF stimulation, but abolishes the response to stimulation of the MT (ITP cooling produced a baseline shift of +5 mV). The MT-evoked response returned to its control value 3 min following cessation of ITP cooling. Calibration: 200 $\mu$V; 5 sec.

of the $R_{VA}$ cells and the accompanying positive SP shift recorded extracellularly. High-frequency stimulation of MT during the blockade was ineffective in eliciting SPs in $R_{VA}$ (fig. 9, Cool ITP or FC), a finding which suggests that MT-evoked positive SPs in $R_{VA}$ are mediated by a pathway involving *both* the FC and the MRF. In contrast to the effects of medial thalamic stimulation, MRF stimulation during ITP blockade elicited a further positive SP in $R_{VA}$ (fig. 9, Cool ITP), although no further shifts were seen in frontal cortex. Thus, it appears that MRF inhibition on R is a direct effect, whereas MT inhibitory effects on R, though they may be indirectly mediated by the MRF, require in addition, the integrity of connections between the FC and R.

*2. SPs accompanying 'Attentive' behavior.* In chronic preparations, sudden unexpected stimuli (doors opening, pencils dropped, etc.) frequently elicited SPs in FC, $R_{VA}$, and MRF (fig. 7, 10C) that were almost identical in time course, amplitude, and polarity to those elicited by MRF stimulation. These SPs appeared to be correlated temporally with a behavioral orienting response. The behavioral and SP responses habituated rapidly. Mildly noxious shocks to the skin elicited similar SPs in FC,

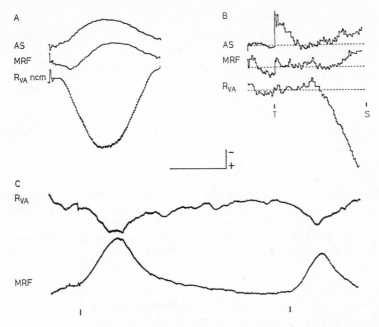

*Fig. 10.* SPs in FC (medial AS), MRF, and nucleus reticularis thalami ($R_{VA}$) evoked by high-frequency medial thalamic (nucleus centralis medialis, ncm) stimulation, conditioned stimuli, and novel stimuli. *A* 15-trial averages of responses to 250-msec, 250-Hz stimulation of medial thalamus (ncm). Surface-negative potentials in FC (AS) and negative potentials in the MRF are accompanied by a larger positive shift in $R_{VA}$. *B* 15-trial averages of responses to a warning tone (T) followed in 6 sec by a noxious skin shock (S); following the tone, negative shifts in FC (AS) and MRF are seen, together with a positive shift in $R_{VA}$. *C* Segment from a continuous recording, showing a negative potential in the MRF accompanying a positive potential in $R_{VA}$ elicited by a sudden noise (first mark). Several seconds later, similar potentials are seen arising spontaneously; these were accompanied by behavioral signs of attentiveness, i.e. the animal raised her head (second mark) from a quiet resting posture and looked around the laboratory for several seconds before again resuming a quiet pose as the SP returned to baseline. Calibration: *A* 1,000 $\mu$V, 4 sec; *B* 200 $\mu$V, 4 sec; *C* 2,000 $\mu$V, 20 sec.

MRF, and $R_{VA}$, but these responses habituated at a slower rate than the SPs accompanying the sound-evoked orienting responses.

SPs in $R_{VA}$, FC, and MRF – similar to those evoked by high frequency MRF or MT stimulation (fig. 10A) or those accompanying orienting responses (fig. 10C) – can be obtained in a conditioning paradigm that creates a state of expectancy (fig. 10B). These conditioned SPs are *not* mani-

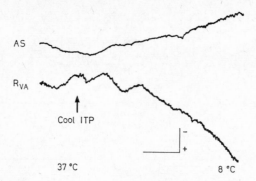

*Fig. 11.* SPs produced in FC (medial AS) and nucleus reticularis thalami ($R_{VA}$) by blockade of the ITP. Onset of cooling (arrow) elicited a slow surface-negative shift in AS and a positive shift in $R_{VA}$; both potentials maintained a tonic level during 10 min of blockade, and returned toward the original levels as the tissue rewarmed following cessation of cooling. Calibration: 1,000 $\mu$V; 10 sec.

fested *in either thalamus or cortex* during ITP blockade [SKINNER and YINGLING, 1976, this volume]. This finding suggests that the mechanism involved in the generation of the cortical and subcortical SPs in response to extrinsic stimuli of behavioral significance involves an interaction between both thalamic and cortical components of the MTFCS.

To summarize the results of this section, positive SP shifts in $R_{VA}$, presumably reflecting inhibition of R units, as well as parallel negative shifts in FC and in the MRF, are elicited by direct MRF stimulation or high frequency MT stimulation. Similar SP shifts accompany orienting responses to novel or noxious stimuli. These SP responses can be conditioned, but the conditioned SPs are manifested only if the functional integrity of the MTFCS is maintained. Thus, it appears that SP shifts in R accompanying conditioned or 'attentive' behavioral states, and presumably reflecting significant changes in thalamocortical gating produced by changes in R unit activity reflected in the SPs, are the result of integration in R of inputs from the MRF and MTFC systems.

## Discussion

The data reported here suggest that nucleus reticularis thalami (R) forms a topographically organized inhibitory feedback mechanism that is capable of controlling patterns of input to the cerebral cortex from all

areas of the thalamus. By controlling cortical input, R would exert a pro-
found influence on the distribution of cortical activity and is thus an obvious candidate for inclusion in any proposed control mechanism in the
brain that underlies functions such as 'attention', in which the concept of
selective control is of central importance.

### A. Regulation of Sensory Evoked Potential Amplitude

Attempts to find a neural basis for modulation of EP amplitude as a
function of 'attention' in both animals and man have been largely unsatis-
factory. The notion of peripheral gating in the sensory pathway as a
mechanism for 'attention' does not provide a ready explanation [cf.
WORDEN, 1966; DESMEDT, 1975; HILLYARD and PICTON, this series]. Our
observations that stimulation of appropriate regions of R can inhibit
selectively transmission through specific thalamic relay nuclei, resulting in
total or near-total abolition of the cortical EP for the specific sensory modality involved provide new evidence for a special form of sensory switching at the thalamic level; this mechanism itself appears to be regulated by
both a higher MTFCS and a lower system, the MRF.

MRF stimulation causes an apparently nonspecific, prolonged enhancement of cortical EPs [DUMONT and DELL, 1960; DESMEDT, 1960].
Since MRF stimulation produces inhibition of R units with a time course
similar to that of the cortical EP facilitation, we suggest that the enhancement of sensory EPs by MRF stimulation is due to a generalized decrease
in the tonic firing rate of inhibitory R neurons that are known to project
onto the thalamic relay nuclei. EPSPs in thalamic relay cells following
MRF stimulation have also been reported [PURPURA et al., 1966 b], but
these potentials are only a few msec in duration; hence, the prolonged facilitation of cortical EPs is more likely to result from removal of thalamic
inhibition originating in R.

While the control of the thalamic gates in R by the MRF seems to
function in a nonselective, generalized manner, the influence of the
MTFCS on R may be quite specific in its operation. Graded cryogenic
blockade of the ITP, which interconnects MT and FC, can produce selective effects on EP amplitude in different sensory modalities [SKINNER and
LINDSLEY, 1971], a finding which suggests that topographical organization, with respect to sensory modalities, exists within this system. Stimulation of FC evokes short-latency excitatory responses in R [WASZAK et al.,
1970; SCHLAG and WASZAK, 1971; STERIADE and WYZINSKI, 1972]. In contrast, ITP blockade produces large positive SP shifts in $R_{VA}$ that are corre-

lated with the inhibition of R units. These results suggest that the FC supplies a tonic excitatory input to R. Functional blockade of the ITP would remove this excitation, lowering the tonic firing rate of R cells and thus reducing their inhibitory effect on specific thalamic nuclei, thereby causing an enhancement of the cortical EP. The apparent topographical organization in the ITP suggests that R could function as the final common pathway in a system for selective gating of thalamocortical activities by the MTFCS.

The MTFCS regulation of R may not be the whole story on the selective regulation of R gates. The presence of local circuit inputs to R (i.e. from a given sense modality) also provides a substrate for selective control of input to a given cortical region. This local regulation of an R gate may be related to 'filtering' or 'selection' processes within that local sense modality itself.

The possibility of selective versus generalized control of R gating functions by the MTFCS and MRF, respectively, thus implies that mechanisms underlying selective perception and generalized arousal may both utilize the same thalamo-cortical gating mechanism. The phylogenetically older MRF appears to have first priority in control of R, as the effects of MRF activation are independent of the MTFCS (fig. 9) and indeed are capable of overriding MTFCS effects (fig. 2); i.e. simultaneous MRF activation (inhibitory on R) and low frequency MT stimulation (excitatory on R) results in inhibition rather than excitation of R units. Thus, a novel stimulus, by activating the MRF, leads to a general inhibition of R, which in effect opens the gates and allows transmission of information about all aspects of the sensory environment to reach the cortex. This overriding effect erases any previously existing pattern of transmission that was established in an earlier behavioral context, and ongoing behavior is interrupted and replaced by a process of scanning of the total sensory environment in order to evaluate the significance of the new stimulus. The evaluation process then results in the establishment of a new pattern of inhibition appropriate to the altered context as the MRF activation subsides. The establishment of a new pattern of selective inhibition, via selective activation of R, is apparently a function of the MTFCS, for: (1) only the MTFCS shows specific sensory regulation, and (2) blockade of the system by lesion of the frontal lobes prevents the subject from ever selectively terminating evoked orienting reactions [LURIA and HOMSKAYA, 1970]. Thus, a mechanism can be envisioned whereby generalized arousal, perhaps corresponding to WILLIAM JAMES' 'reflexive attention', would involve *generalized inhibition* of R (and hence disinhibition of thalamo-cortical pathways) as a result of activation of the MRF, while selective attention would result from precisely organized patterns of inhibition originating in the MTFCS and expressed via *patterned activation* of R.

How patterns of activity arising in $R_{VA}$ under MTFCS control could be transmitted to more lateral and posterior regions of R adjacent to thalamic relay nuclei remains enigmatic. Approximately 10% of R cell axons remain within the confines of R, and the major source of input to a given R cell appears to be from other R cells [SCHEIBEL and SCHEIBEL, 1966], However, more posterior and lateral regions of R exhibit a striking scarcity of presynaptic neuropil and dendritic spines when compared with $R_{VA}$, and instead tightly packed bundles of parallel R cell dendrites are seen [SCHEIBEL and SCHEIBEL, 1972]. Dendro-dendritic synaptic interactions may perhaps play a role in transmission and processing of information in areas of R posterior to the anterior neuropil region of $R_{VA}$.

The possibility for either generalized or specific control of R, coupled with its unique capacity to influence all thalamocortical activities, suggests that R is an integrative control mechanism which influences EP phenomena and also such high order functions as differential states of consciousness or selective attention.

### B. Regulation of Synchronous Activity

Synchronous activity in the 8–12 Hz range (the 'alpha' rhythm of the EEG) has been associated with inattentive states since the early studies of BERGER [1929]. The unit recordings from $R_{VA}$ reported here suggest that inhibitory gating activities originating in R play a key role in the generation of this rhythmicity, and once again an interplay between MRF and MTFCS effects on R seems to be of crucial importance.

Medial thalamic stimulation producing RRs [MORISON and DEMPSEY, 1942] has been shown to produce prolonged IPSPs in VL relay cells [PURPURA and COHEN, 1962]. During these IPSPs, cerebellar input to VL no longer elicits the usual monosynaptic response [PURPURA et al., 1965], a result which has been interpreted as 'functional deafferentation of motor cortex elements' [PURPURA, 1970]. Several workers [SCHLAG and WASZAK, 1970, 1971; FILION et al., 1971; FRIGYESI, 1971, 1972; FRIGYESI and SCHWARTZ, 1972; LAMARRE et al., 1971] have noted an inverse relationship between the unit activity in R and VL. This relation suggests that inhibitory projections from R may produce the phasic IPSPs in VL, the classical motor relay nucleus. WASZAK [1972, 1973, 1974] has argued, however, that VL inhibition originating in R may be tonic rather than phasic in character, but the question of the phasic versus tonic nature of R inhibition of VL must be regarded as still unsettled. This question may contain an oversimplified notion about the relationship, however, because the extensive branching of R cell axons suggests that terminals from several R cells could converge upon a single VL cell so that the IPSPs produced in the VL cell would depend on the summated activity in a population of R cells, whose pattern might not always be reflected in a single-unit recording.

The situation is clearer for the RR elicited by a series of regularly timed stimuli. Our results favor the interpretation of a direct relationship between bursts of firing in R and individual IPSPs during the RR. Supporting this view are the facts that (1) latencies of R bursts to MT stimulation (0–30 msec) agree well with the range of latencies (15–40 msec) reported for IPSPs in VL [PURPURA and COHEN, 1962]; (2) the frequency and duration of R bursts increase with each successive stimulus, closely paralleling the cortical recruiting response; (3) the PST histograms of R bursts mirror the reported waveforms of phasic thalamic IPSPs, and (4) simultaneous MRF stimulation, which abolishes both the cortical response and the thalamic IPSPs [PURPURA et al., 1966b], also prevents the response of R cells to MT stimulation. This last observation provides an obvious explanation for EEG desynchronization by the MRF. Any activation of the MRF by electrical or behavioral stimuli results in rapid and prolonged inhibition of $R_{VA}$ units. During MRF activation, R cells can no longer fire in response to MT stimulation. The gating IPSPs which R units produce in thalamic relay nuclei are thus abolished, RRs or spontaneously occurring rhythmic activity are blocked, and afferent input to the cortex is restored.

Orbitofrontal cortex lesions [VELASCO et al., 1968] and lesions or cryogenic blockade of ITP [SKINNER and LINDSLEY, 1967], abolish RRs in the thalamus as well as in the cortex. In this present study, ITP blockade abolished in parallel the RRs and the burst responses of $R_{VA}$ cells to MT stimulation, a finding which suggests that activation of $R_{VA}$ units during RRs requires a descending influence from FC via the ITP. Since no cells have been recorded in FC with the long-burst properties presumably necessary for production of prolonged IPSPs (assuming no prolonged transmitter action), we think that R cell (and not FC cell) bursts are responsible for the thalamic IPSPs underlying RRs.

At least two possible mechanisms could explain the effect of ITP blockade on $R_{VA}$ unit responses: (1) activation of R cells is via a pathway from MT to FC and back to R via the ITP, or (2) the FC supplies a tonic facilitatory input to R which is necessary for R units to respond to a direct MT-R activation. Intracellular recordings from R units during ITP blockade may be necessary to resolve the issue, but several indirect lines of evidence favor the first alternative. First, the observation that ITP blockade prevents the occurrence of SPs as well as unit responses in $R_{VA}$ to MT stimulation implies that MT effects on $R_{VA}$ are mediated via FC. The latency of the $R_{VA}$ unit responses to MT stimulation (10–30 msec) is compatible with a long thalamo-cortico-R pathway. DESIRAJU and PUR-PURA [1970], reporting on reciprocal production of IPSPs in MT and VL to stimulation of VL and MT, respectively, note that VL-evoked IPSPs in MT cells have a short latency of 1.5–4.0 msec, whereas the latency of MT-evoked responses in VL cells is 15–40 msec. They attribute this difference to differences in complexity in the reciprocal thalamic pathways. Our results show that the unit responses in $R_{VA}$ to MT stimulation could underlie production of the long-latency IPSPs in VL. However, the same $R_{VA}$ cells which fire long bursts to MT stimulation do not respond to stimulation of VL, and hence are not involved in production of the short-latency IPSPs in MT. Thus, we suggest that MT-evoked IPSPs in VL are produced by an MT-FC-R pathway. VL-evoked IPSPs in MT cells are produced by a much shorter pathway not involving R and probably mediated by inhibitory interneurons within the thalamus itself.

SCHLAG and VILLABLANCA [1967] have suggested using the term incrementing activity for both RRs and ARs, since in each case, biphasic positive-negative waveforms are recorded in the primary projection cortex of the thalamic nucleus being stimulated, and monophasic negative waveforms are seen in surrounding cortical areas. However, SKINNER and LINDSLEY [1973] favored retaining the distinction between RRs and ARs, since stimulation of medial thalamic nuclei has different effects on behavior than stimulation of the lateral (specific) nuclei.

Our present results suggest, however, that in addition to the behavioral distinction, there is a fundamental difference in the neuronal mechanisms involved in the generation of RRs and ARs so that we propose the retention of both terms. RRs are produced by stimulation of medial thalamic nuclei, and involve the generation of thalamic IPSPs by a mechanism involving FC and R. ARs are produced by stimulation of lateral thalamic nuclei, and involve the generation of thalamic IPSPs by a wholly intrinsic thalamic mechanism that does not include R.

Pulsed input to deafferented cortex results in incrementing wave activity [SCHLAG and VILLABLANCA, 1967], although such rhythmic activity is not normally seen in isolated cortex. Hence, it appears that rhythmically pulsed input is necessary and sufficient for the production of cortical rhythmicity. Spindle-like activity can be observed in the thalamus after total decortication [VILLABLANCA and SCHLAG, 1968], an observation which has led to the conclusion that the pacemaker for rhythmic cortical activity is located within the thalamus. However, results from sequential lesions of different cortical areas [VELASCO and LINDSLEY, 1965; VELASCO et al., 1968] suggest that this may be an oversimplified notion. Removal of most sensory and association areas of cortex increases the amplitude of spontaneous spindle waves. However, removal of a limited area of orbitofrontal cortex totally abolishes spindles in both thalamus and cortex, an effect that is reversed by further total decortication. This observation, together with the fact that lesions or cryogenic blockade of the ITP [SKINNER and LINDSLEY, 1967] also abolish recruiting responses (RRs) and spindles, suggests that the orbitofrontal cortex, together with the medial thalamus, form part of a system normally involved in the generation of rhythmic activity in other parts of the thalamus and cortex. The rhythmic activity observed in the thalamus after total decortication may reflect the activity of intrathalamic elements related to the production of ARs by stimulation of VL. The VL stimulation activates shorter-latency pathways apparently not involving R, and hence not dependent on a cortical pathway for their activation. This interpretation is supported by findings that ARs are not affected by ITP blockade [SKINNER and LINDSLEY, 1967; SKINNER, 1971b].

Working within these constraints, it is possible to suggest a plausible sequence of events in the production of RRs. Medial thalamic stimulation activates a rostrally conducting pathway running through the ITP and excites an area of the FC. This excitation is reflected in the initial surface-positive wave of the biphasic RR, which is only recorded in this region [SCHLAG and VILLABLANCA, 1967]. Subsequent to this excitation, both the FC and large areas of surrounding cortex are subject to prolonged inhibition which is reflected in the surface-negative component of the RR. Meanwhile, activity from the FC is transmitted back through the ITP and excites cells in $R_{VA}$, causing them to fire prolonged bursts which inhibit cells of VL and perhaps other thalamic relay nuclei. These R bursts may inhibit MT cells as well, since MT cells also show long-latency, prolonged IPSPs during RRs [PURPURA and SHOFER, 1963]. The period of cortical inhibition corresponds in latency and duration to the period of thalamic inhibition, and if the next stimulus is timed to occur during the following period of rebound excitation, the response in both thalamus and cortex increments, resulting in the recruiting character of the response. The net result of this process is to suppress the activity of involved areas of cortex by removing the thalamic input at the same time that the cortex itself is inhibited. The operation of this dual-level control mechanism is also reflected in the reduction of EP amplitudes, which decrease as the amplitude of the RR increases [JASPER and AJMONE-MARSAN, 1952].

### C. Regulation of Slow Potential Activity in Cortex

The discovery of the contingent negative variation (CNV) by WALTER et al. [1964] has created much interest in SP shifts as possible correlates of attention, arousal, and expectancy. Our animal studies have shown that a surface-negative, depth-positive cortical shift, localized to frontal regions, accompanies orienting responses and states of conditioned expectancy (fig. 7, 10b). This negative cortical shift is accompanied by a large positive shift in $R_{VA}$ and parts of $R_{VL}$ which can reach several mV in amplitude. SP shifts in both FC and R, virtually identical to those elicited by novel stimuli, can be elicited by electrical stimulation of the MRF (fig. 7), a finding which suggests that MRF activation may play a major role in the initiation of these SPs. This interpretation is further supported by DC recordings from the MRF, which show negative SPs (presumably reflecting excitation of MRF units) paralleling the SPs in FC and R (fig. 10b, c).

High frequency stimulation of the MT produces SPs in FC and R similar to those evoked by MRF stimulation; such MT stimuli also evoke negative SPs in the MRF (fig. 10a), a finding which further supports the suggestion that MRF activation is the primary event responsible for evoking the SPs in FC and R. In the example shown, the negative SP in MRF appears to have a somewhat longer latency than the positive SP in $R_{VA}$. This, however, does not preclude the interpretation that MRF activation precedes the events in R, since (1) the slow onset of SPs makes precise latency measurements difficult; (2) electrode drift or baseline shifts unrelated to the evoked activity may obscure lower amplitude early components of the response; (3) the exact mechanism of generation of the SPs is unknown, and may involve passive participation of glial elements [LOTHMAN and SOMJEN, 1975], and (4) imprecise placement of electrodes outside the center of a slowly spreading focus of activity could result in misleading interpretations of latency data.

While the desynchronizing effect of high frequency MT stimulation appears to be mediated by an MT-MRF pathway, as lesions behind the MT abolish the effect [SCHLAG and CHAILLET, 1963], our results suggest that the FC may also be involved in this phenomenon, since ITP blockade abolishes the positive SP in R produced by high frequency MT stimulation (fig. 9). A possible anatomical substrate for this phenomenon might be the FC-MRF connection described by NAUTA [1964]. The fact that SP responses in R to MRF stimulation remain intact during ITP blockade (fig. 9) indicates again that the MRF is probably the final link in the pathway for production of these SPs. SCHEIBEL and SCHEIBEL [1966] traced fibers from the MRF running through subthalamic and hypothalamic areas into ventral regions of $R_{VA}$ as well as more lateral regions of R; this provides a likely pathway for mediation of the MRF-induced SP shifts in R as well as the inhibitory effects of the MRF on R unit activity.

Aversive conditioning experiments have shown that a state of expectancy elicited by a tone preceding an unavoidable noxious shock is accompanied by SPs in FC, MRF, and R, all of which are virtually identical to those produced by MRF activation (fig. 10b) [for further discussion, see SKINNER and YINGLING, this volume]. Blockade of the MTFCS abolishes the SPs in both R and FC, but it is not known whether or not the effect of ITP blockade is mediated via the MRF. Since MRF stimulation can still produce positive SPs in $R_{VA}$ during ITP blockade (fig. 9), it may be that the abolition of conditioned SPs in R reflects a failure of the conditioned stimulus to activate the MRF during the blockade. A possible alternative is that convergent influences from FC and MRF are both required to elicit the conditioned SPs in R.

While many questions remain unanswered at this time, it is nevertheless apparent that many SP phenomena associated with attention are the result of complex interactions between the MRF, MTFCS, and R, structures which also interact as parts of one complex system to regulate synchronous spontaneous cortical activity and EP amplitude.

## Summary

Recordings of slow potentials (SPs), evoked potentials (EPs), and unit responses have been employed to investigate the functioning of nucleus reticularis thalami (R) and its control by the mediothalamic-frontocortical system (MTFCS) and the mesencephalic reticular formation (MRF). Stimulation of a given region of R can selectively control the amplitude of EPs transmitted through the adjacent specific relay nucleus without affecting transmission through the other relay nuclei. Inhibitory projections from cells in R appear to underlie the prolonged phasic IPSPs recorded in the thalamus during 8–12 Hz synchronous activity.

Novel or conditioned stimuli evoke large positive SPs in R which are associated with unit inhibition and a removal of the R inhibitory control of thalamo-cortical pathways. Activities in R are subject to *generalized inhibitory* control by the MRF and *selective excitatory* modulation by the MTFCS. It is interpreted that the MRF-MTFC-R system, by regulating information processing in other areas of the brain, may underlie the phenomenon of attention.

## Acknowledgments

This work was supported by Grants HL 13837 and HL 17907 from the National Heart and Lung Institute, NIH, USPHS. C. D. YINGLING was a National Science Foundation Graduate Fellow. The assistance of GREGORY L. KING is greatly appreciated.

## References

BERGER, H.: Über das Elektrenkephalogramm des Menschen. Arch. Psychiat. Nerv-Krankh. *87:* 527–570 (1929).

CARMAN, J. B.; COWAN, W. M., and POWELL, T. P. S.: Cortical connexions of the thalamic reticular nucleus. J. Anat. *98:* 587–598 (1964).

CHOW, K. L.: Regional degeneration of the thalamic reticular nucleus following cortical ablations in the monkey. J. comp. Neurol. *97:* 37–59 (1952).

DESIRAJU, T. and PURPURA, D. P.: Organization of specific-nonspecific thalamic internuclear synaptic pathways. Brain Res. *21:* 169–181 (1970).

DESMEDT, J. E.: Neurophysiological mechanisms controlling acoustic input; in RASMUSSEN and WINDLE Neural mechanisms of the auditory and vestibular systems, pp. 152–164 (Thomas, Springfield 1960).

DESMEDT, J. E.: Physiological studies of the efferent recurrent auditory system; in KEIDEL and NEFF Handbook of sensory physiology, vol. 5, part 2, chap. 5, pp. 219–246 (Springer, Berlin 1975).

DUMONT, S. et DELL, P.: Facilitation réticulaire des mécanismes visuels corticaux. Electroenceph. clin. Neurophysiol. *12:* 769–796 (1960).

FILION, M.; LAMARRE, Y., and CORDEAU, J. P.: Neuronal discharges of the ventrolateral nucleus of the thalamus during sleep and wakefulness in the cat. II. Evoked activity. Expl Brain Res. *12:* 499–508 (1971).

FRIGYESI, T. L.: Organization of synaptic pathways linking the head of the caudate nucleus to the dorsal thalamus. Int. J. Neurol. *8:* 111–138 (1971).

FRIGYESI, T. L.: Intracellular recordings from neurons in dorsolateral thalamic reticular nucleus during capsular, basal ganglia, and midline thalamic stimulation. Brain Res. *48:* 157–172 (1972).

FRIGYESI, T. L. and SCHWARTZ, R.: Cortical control of thalamic sensori-motor relay activities in the cat and the squirrel monkey; in FRIGYESI, RINVIK and YAHR Corticothalamic projections and sensorimotor activities, pp. 161–195 (Raven Press, Hewlett 1972).

JASPER, H. H.: Diffuse projection systems. The integrative action of the thalamic reticular system. Electroenceph. clin. Neurophysiol. *1:* 405–420 (1949).

JASPER, H. H. and AJMONE-MARSAN, C.: Thalamo-cortical integrating mechanisms. Res. Publ. Ass. nerv. ment. Dis. *30:* 493–512 (1952).

JASPER, H. H. and AJMONE-MARSAN, C.: A stereotaxic atlas of the diencephalon of the cat (National Research Council of Canada, Ottawa 1954).

JONES, E. G.: Some aspects of the organization of the thalamic reticular complex. J. comp. Neurol. *162:* 295–308 (1975).

LAMARRE, Y.; FILION, M., and CORDEAU, J. P.: Neuronal discharges of the ventrolateral nucleus of the thalamus during sleep and wakefulness in the cat. I. Spontaneous activity. Expl Brain Res. *12:* 480–498 (1971).

LOTHMAN, E. W. and SOMJEN, G. G.: Extracellular potassium activity, intracellular and extracellular potential responses in the spinal cord. J. Physiol., Lond. *252:* 115–136 (1975).

LURIA, A. R. and HOMSKAYA, E. D.: Frontal lobes and the regulation of arousal processes; in MOSTOFSKY Attention: contemporary theory and analysis, pp. 303–330 (Appleton Century Crofts, New York 1970).

MORISON, R. S. and DEMPSEY, E. W.: A study of thalamocortical relations. Am. J. Physiol. *135:* 281–292 (1942).

NAUTA, W. J. H.: Some efferent connections of the prefrontal cortex in the monkey; in WARREN and AKERT The frontal granular cortex and behavior, pp. 397–409 (McGraw-Hill, New York 1964).

PURPURA, D. P.: Operations and processes in thalamic and synaptically related neural subsystems; in SCHMITT The neurosciences: second study program, pp. 458–470 (Rockefeller University Press, New York 1970).

PURPURA, D. P. and COHEN, B.: Intracellular recording from thalamic neurons during recruiting responses. J. Neurophysiol. *25:* 621–635 (1962).

PURPURA, D. P.; FRIGYESI, T. L.; MCMURTRY, J. G., and SCARFF, T.: Synaptic mechanisms in thalamic regulation of cerebello-cortical projection activity; in PURPURA and YAHR The thalamus, pp. 153–172 (Columbia University Press, New York 1966a).

PURPURA, D. P.; MCMURTRY, J. G., and MAEKAWA, K.: Synaptic events in ventrolateral thalamic neurons during suppression of recruiting responses by brain stem reticular stimulation. Brain Res. *1:* 63–76 (1966b).

PURPURA, D. P.; SCARFF, T., and MCMURTRY, J. G.: Intracellular study of internuclear inhibition in ventrolateral thalamic neurons. J. Neurophysiol. *28:* 487–496 (1965).

PURPURA, D. P. and SHOFER, R. J.: Intracellular recording from thalamic neurons during reticulocortical activation. J. Neurophysiol. *26:* 494–505 (1963).

RAMÓN Y CAJAL, S.: Histologie du système nerveux de l'homme et des vertébrés, vol. 1 and 2 (Maloine, Paris 1909/1911).

Rose, J. E.: The cortical connections of the reticular complex of the thalamus. Res. Publ. Ass. nerv. ment. Dis. *30:* 454–479 (1952).

Rose, J. E. and Woolsey, C. N.: Organization of the mammalian thalamus and its relationships to the cerebral cortex. Electroenceph. clin. Neurophysiol. *1:* 391–404 (1949).

Scheibel, M. E. and Scheibel, A. B.: The organization of the nucleus reticularis thalami. A Golgi study. Brain Res. *1:* 43–62 (1966).

Scheibel, M. E. and Scheibel, A. B.: Structural organization of non-specific thalamic nuclei and their projection toward cortex. Brain Res. *6:* 60–94 (1967).

Scheibel, M. E. and Scheibel, A. B.: Specialized organizational patterns within the nucleus reticularis thalami of the cat. Expl Neurol. *34:* 316–322 (1972).

Schlag, J.: Reactions and interactions to stimulation of the motor cortex of the cat. J. Neurophysiol. *29:* 44–71 (1966).

Schlag, J. and Balvin, R.: Sequence of events following synaptic and electrical excitation of pyramidal neurons of the motor cortex. J. Neurophysiol. *27:* 334–365 (1964).

Schlag, J. D. and Chaillet, F.: Thalamic mechanisms involved in cortical desynchronization and recruiting responses. Electroenceph. clin. Neurophysiol. *15:* 39–62 (1963).

Schlag, J. and Villablanca, J.: Cortical incremental responses to thalamic stimulation. Brain Res. *6:* 119–142 (1967).

Schlag, J. and Waszak, M.: Characteristics of unit responses in nucleus reticularis thalami. Brain Res. *21:* 286–288 (1970).

Schlag, J. and Waszak, M.: Electrophysiological properties of units of the thalamic reticular complex. Expl Neurol. *32:* 79–97 (1971).

Skinner, J. E.: Neuroscience. A laboratory manual (Saunders, Philadelphia 1971a).

Skinner, J. E.: Abolition of several forms of cortical synchronization during blockade in the inferior thalamic peduncle. Electroenceph. clin. Neurophysiol. *31:* 211–221 (1971b).

Skinner, J. E. and Lindsley, D. B.: Electrophysiological and behavioral effects of blockade of the nonspecific thalamo-cortical system. Brain Res. *6:* 95–118 (1967).

Skinner, J. E. and Lindsley, D. B.: Enhancement of visual and auditory evoked potentials during blockade of the non-specific thalamo-cortical system. Electroenceph. clin. Neurophysiol. *31:* 1–6 (1971).

Skinner, J. E. and Yingling, C. D.: Regulation of slow potential shifts in nucleus reticularis thalami by the mesencephalic reticular formation and the frontal granular cortex. Electroenceph. clin. Neurophysiol. *40:* 288–296 (1976).

Steriade, M. and Wyzinski, P.: Cortically elicited activities in thalamic reticularis neurons. Brain Res. *42:* 514–520 (1972).

Velasco, M. and Lindsley, D. B.: Role of orbital cortex in regulation of thalamo-cortical electrical activity. Science *149:* 1375–1377 (1965).

Velasco, M.; Skinner, J. E.; Asaro, K. D., and Lindsley, D. B.: Thalamo-cortical systems regulating spindle bursts and recruiting responses. I. Effect of cortical ablations. Electroenceph. clin. Neurophysiol. *25:* 463–470 (1968).

VILLABLANCA, J. and SCHLAG, J.: Cortical control of thalamic spindle waves. Expl Neurol. *20:* 432–442 (1968).

WALTER, W. G.; COOPER, R.; ALDRIDGE, V. J.; McCALLUM, W. C., and WINTER, A. L.: Contingent negative variation: an electric sign of sensori-motor association and expectancy in the human brain. Nature, Lond. *203:* 380–384 (1964).

WASZAK, M.: Membrane potential changes in rostral thalamic neurons during spontaneous and triggered spindles. Brain Res. *41:* 479–481 (1972).

WASZAK, M.: Effect of polarizing currents on potentials evoked in neurons of the ventral leaf of nucleus reticularis thalami by intralaminar stimulation. Expl Neurol. *40:* 82–89 (1973).

WASZAK, M.: Effect of barbiturate anesthesia on discharge pattern in nucleus reticularis thalami. Pharmac. biochem. Behav. *2:* 339–345 (1974).

WASZAK, M.; SCHLAG, J. D., and FEENEY, D. M.: Thalamic incremental responses to prefrontal cortical stimulation in the cat. Brain Res. *21:* 105–113 (1970).

WORDEN, F. G.: Attention and auditory electrophysiology; in STELLAR and SPRAGUE Progress in physiological psychology, vol. 1, pp. 45–116 (Academic Press, New York 1966).

YINGLING, C. D. and SKINNER, J. E.: Regulation of unit activity in nucleus reticularis thalami by the mesencephalic reticular formation and the frontal granular cortex. Electroenceph. clin. Neurophysiol. *39:* 635–642 (1975).

YINGLING, C. D. and SKINNER, J. E.: Selective regulation of thalamic sensory relay nuclei by nucleus reticularis thalami. Electroenceph. clin. Neurophysiol. *41:* 476–482 (1976).

Dr. CHARLES D. YINGLING, Langley Porter Neuropsychiatric Institute, University of California, 401 Parnassus Avenue, *San Francisco, CA 94143* (USA). Tel. (415) 681 8080.

Prof. JAMES E. SKINNER, Neurophysiology Section, Physiology Department, Baylor Medical College, Texas Medical Center, *Houston, TX 77030* (USA). Tel. (713) 790 3105.

Attention, Voluntary Contraction and Event-Related Cerebral Potentials.
Prog. clin. Neurophysiol., vol. 1, Ed. J. E. DESMEDT, pp. 97–131 (Karger, Basel 1977)

# Motor and Sensory Determinants of Cortical Slow Potential Shifts in Man[1]

KARL SYNDULKO and DONALD B. LINDSLEY

Gateways Hospital and University of California, Los Angeles, Calif.

## I. Introduction

Brain electrical activity, when recorded at the scalp under appropriate conditions and with suitable time-constants, may reveal three major categories of electrical potentials: (1) electroencephalogram (EEG) – continuous, often rhythmic, potential fluctuations ranging in frequency from less than 1 to 50 or 60 cps; (2) evoked potentials (EPs) – discrete potential fluctuations of variable frequency and limited duration (typically less than 500 msec) which occur only in response to presented or expected sensory stimuli, or which are associated with emitted contractions; and (3) slow potential shifts (SPSs) – low frequency (<1 cps) potentials that reflect changes in state or that occur preparatory to stimulus input or motor output. The separation of scalp electrocortical activity into 3 categories does not imply complete independence of the different types of potentials. Independence should be demonstrated empirically.

The present study is concerned with SPSs and the contingent negative variation (CNV) as a special class of SPSs. For the purposes of this paper, a SPS is defined as a low frequency positive or negative change in the resting, EEG potential level that has a minimum period of a few hundred milliseconds and a maximum period of less than 10 sec, that is closely related to specifiable stimulus or behavioral events, and that can be reliably elicited under a definable set of conditions. SPSs outside of this definition have been described [O'LEARY and GOLDRING, 1964], but these may involve fundamentally different mechanisms than the SPSs under investigation here and will not be considered further.

[1] This research was supported by NASA Grant NGL 05-007-049 and USPHS Grant NS-8552 to D. B. LINDSLEY.

The CNV was first recorded by WALTER *et al.* [1964]. Their investigations up to 1966 associated the CNV with such psychological processes as attention and expectancy, with cerebral processes preparatory both to overt motor responses and to mental responses or decisions, and had demonstrated the importance of attitude and motivation for the appearance and maintenance of CNV [WALTER, 1967].

Investigations directed at confirmation and extension of WALTER's original findings on the CNV followed in increasing numbers, as is evident in recent reviews [COHEN, 1969; McCALLUM and KNOTT, 1973; TECCE, 1972]. From these studies, it is apparent that the CNV can be recorded in a wide variety of experimental situations, each of which fits commonly employed operational definitions of a number of different psychological processes [McCALLUM and WALTER, 1968; HILLYARD, 1973]. In fact, the behavioral situations accompanied by CNV and the range of experimental manipulations affecting CNV are diverse enough to raise questions as to whether or not the CNV is a unitary process [BORDA, 1970; JARVILEHTO and FRUHSTORFER, 1970; LOW, 1969].

Topographical distribution has been utilized as a means of differentiating EPs [GOFF *et al.*, 1969; VAUGHAN, 1969], but has not been applied frequently and systematically to the study of CNV. In the few studies of CNV that have employed topographical distribution as a dependent variable, changes in CNV topography were obtained to particular experimental manipulations [BORDA, 1970; CANT and BICKFORD, 1967; JARVILEHTO and FRUHSTORFER, 1970]. Results of these studies support the differential contribution of topographically distinct, independent SPS generators in different tasks. Further topographical distribution studies are needed for the CNV and related SPSs recorded in different experimental tasks to distinguish the possible sources of SPSs. In addition, determination of SPS topography in different behavioral tasks may permit a better understanding of the physiological processes involved in those behavioral situations, especially if the distributions can be related to SPSs recorded in animals and to other SPSs recorded in humans.

The present experiments investigate regional differences in SPSs over the surface of the scalp during preparation for the performance of tasks which were designed to emphasize either *sensory* or *motor* components. Two kinds of regional differentiations were examined: (1) lateral SPS differences that might be related to the unilateral response requirements of motor tasks, or to cerebral dominance, and (2) anterior-posterior gradients of potential along the midline, that might be related to the sensory or motor character of the experimental situation. The results of three experiments and an eye movement control procedure are presented below. These are followed by a discussion of the results and by general comments on the functional significance of the SPSs under investigation.

## II. Lateral SPS Differences

The relationship between lateral asymmetries of SPSs and unimanual muscle contractions has been most extensively studied for uncued motor responses. KORNHUBER and DEECKE [1965] and GILDEN et al. [1966] were first to describe a series of response-related components that preceded distal muscle movements. Some of these components appeared to exhibit lateral asymmetry with maximal amplitudes over sensorimotor cortex contralateral to the movement. Although controversy has arisen as to which components show contralateral localization (this volume), it appears that the initial negative SPS preceding uncued movements is at least a few microvolts larger over the contralateral sensorimotor area.

In view of the findings of contralaterally dominant negative SPSs prior to uncued responses, it is surprising that a number of topographical investigations of SPSs, i.e. CNVs, during warned RT tasks have failed to demonstrate comparable response-related asymmetries [for a review, see TECCE, 1972].

The apparent difference in SPS distributions for warned as opposed to unwarned motor responses may reflect fundamentally different cortical preparatory processes for the two classes of responses. On the other hand, the topographical differences may reflect a number of methodological variations in studies of cued versus uncued motor output, such as differential emphasis on unimanual response preparation, degree of response automation, degree of response imperativeness, or even the psychological consequences of the response. In any case, a comparison of the two response modes may have important implications for understanding the functional role of contralateral sensorimotor cortex in response preparation.

Two studies, which were specifically directed at investigating lateral asymmetries over sensorimotor cortex during warned response preparation, have provided evidence that is contradictory to that presented above [OTTO and LEIFER, 1973; SYNDULKO, 1969]. Results of these studies showed that under certain conditions the sensorimotor SPS contralateral to a warned movement is more negative than the ipsilateral SPS, although the differences were small. In order to examine this issue more systematically, we examined the following hypotheses: (1) During a warned reaction time task that permits preparation for a unimanual response, the SPS over cortex contralateral to the response should be larger than that over homologous ipsilateral cortex. (2) The lateral asymmetry obtained in (1) should be largest over sensorimotor cortex if the electrocortical asymmetry represents response-related preparatory activity. (3) The lateral SPS asymmetries obtained in (1) and (2) should not occur during a warning interval that does not require response preparation. (4) Response-related lateral SPS asymmetries should not be observed during a warning interval that requires bimanual response preparation. (5) Lateral SPS asymmetries could be related to cerebral dominance as determined by hand preference.

### Method

Subjects were 9 right-handed and 5 left-handed college students. Handedness was determined by a short questionnaire adopted from Hécaen and Ajuriaguerra [1964]. Three experimental conditions were employed in one 2-hour session, with the order of conditions counterbalanced among Ss. In the specific warning (SW) task the warning signal (S1) was a 50-msec oscilloscopic display of either the word LEFT or RIGHT. After an interstimulus interval (ISI) of 1.5 sec, the same word was presented at S2 and the S was required to make an appropriate left or right index finger extension (R). 15 presentations of each of the two types of trials (S1-S2-R) were randomly intermixed in a series in order to control for tonic preparatory sets based on expected left or right-hand response trials. Except for the random intermixture of left and right-response trials, the SW task is similar to the simple warned reaction time tasks typically used in CNV studies. It was expected the SPS asymmetries would develop during the S1-S2 interval and that, in accordance with hypothesis 1, the direction of asymmetry would be dependent on the side of unimanual preparation.

The general warning (GW) condition was a warned disjunctive reaction time task. S1 was the word BOTH, the ISI was 1.5 sec, and S2 was either the word LEFT or RIGHT. Ss were instructed to prepare both left and right finger responses at S1 and then to make only the indicated response at S2. In view of the bimanual response preparation required to perform this task, no response-related SPS asymmetries were expected (hypothesis 4). However, it was expected that an inherent lateral SPS asymmetry such as that based on hand preference (presumed cerebral dominance) would manifest itself during GW (hypothesis 5). In both the SW and GW conditions Ss were instructed to respond as fast as possible to S2. Reaction times were measured and immediately fed back visually to provide added incentive for fast responses. Explicit instructions and practice trials were given to insure stable performance.

The visual discrimination (VD) condition involved a visual movement discrimination task. The S watched a 4×4 array of dots which appeared at S1 and remained on for 1,450 msec, whereupon the dot array shifted position either horizontally or vertically. The shifted pattern was S2 and remained on for 50 msec. The S was instructed to report the direction of shift at S3 (the word REPORT presented 1.5 sec after S2) by making a right finger extension for horizontal shifts or a left finger extension for vertical shifts. 16 trials each of horizontal and vertical movements were presented randomly intermixed. Response accuracy, not response speed, was emphasized, and the word CORRECT or WRONG was presented visually immediately after the press to indicate the correctness of the reported discrimination. It was expected that during the S1-S2 interval, which involved preparation for a visual discrimination, response-related SPS asymmetries would not be evident over sensorimotor areas (hypothesis 3). However, such response-related asymmetries were expected during the S2-S3 motor preparatory interval if response speed was not a critical variable.

The experiments were controlled using a PDP-12 computer that presented stimuli and RT feedback on a remote oscilloscope. Bipolar transhemispheric EEG recordings were made at frontal ($F_3$-$F_4$), parietal ($P_3$-$P_4$) and occipital ($O_1$-$O_2$) sites. Recordings were also made at $C_3$ and $C_4$ referenced to linked earlobe electrodes. To obtain the bipolar record, $C_3$-$C_4$, point by point subtractions were made on the PDP-12 between the averaged SPS records at $C_4$ and $C_3$. Although a fixation point was used to minimize eye movements, vertical electro-oculogram (EOG) was monitored continuously. Only trials without eye movement artifacts or response errors were included in the SPS averages. Both EOG and EEG were recorded with Grass DC amplifiers modified for recording with a 12-sec time constant. An upper, $1/2$ amplitude setting of 15 Hz was used to reduce high frequency contamination of the SPSs. Data were recorded on FM magnetic tape for off-line digitizing (62.75 samples/sec/channel) and automatic quantification on the PDP-12. SPSs were quantified by making an average amplitude measure over the 200-msec interval prior to S2 (and S3 where appropriate) relative to the mean voltage level of the 500-msec, pre-S1, baseline interval.

## Results

Figure 1 shows superimposed, grand mean SPSs from left ($C_3$) and right ($C_4$) sensorimotor areas during left- and right-hand response trials of the SW, GW, and VD conditions for both right- and left-handed Ss. It will be noted that for right-handed Ss in the SW condition, pre-S2, SPS amplitude was more negative over the sensorimotor area contralateral to the hand response made after S2. The inter-hemispheric difference in SPS amplitude was greater during preparation for right responses than for left responses. For right response trials, the SPS over the left sensorimotor region became more negative than the homologous right area within a few hundred milliseconds after S1 and remained more negative throughout the S1-S2 warning period and even beyond the time of the motor response to S2. In left response trials, the SPS over $C_3$ was again more neg-

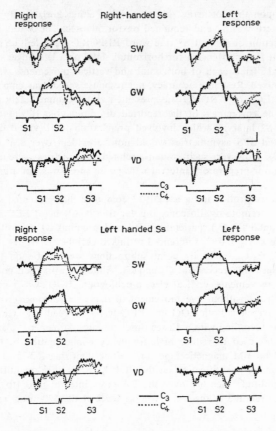

*Fig. 1.* Superimposition of grand mean SPSs at left ($C_3$) and right ($C_4$) sensori-motor cortex for 8 right-handed and 5 left-handed $Ss$. Records were obtained during right-hand and left-hand response trials in the specific warning (SW), general warning (GW) and visual discrimination (VD) conditions. Negativity is up. Calibrations: 500 msec; 10 $\mu$V.

ative immediately after S1, but $C_4$ became more negative about 500 msec before the onset of S2 and the subsequent left-hand response.

In the S1-S2 interval of the GW condition, during which bimanual response preparation was required, inter-hemispheric differences in SPSs were not apparent, at least immediately before S2. The absence of preparation for a unimanual response was thus paralleled by the absence of pre-S2 differences in SPSs over left and right sensorimotor areas. However, inter-hemispheric differences in potential level did occur in the period immediately after S1 and after S2, and these SPS differences were in the same direction as those in the SW condition for the corresponding periods. Thus, the major differences in SPS laterality at $C_3$ and $C_4$ between the SW and GW conditions occurred during the pre-S2 motor preparatory interval. In SW, there was unimanual response preparation and inter-hemispheric SPS differences occurred, while in GW bimanual response preparation was required and comparable pre-response differences did not occur.

Inter-hemispheric differences in SPSs also occurred during the VD condition, but were most prominent during the S2-S3 interval. The S2-S3 interval was similar to the S1-S2 interval of the SW condition, in that both required preparation for a specific motor response. Likewise, the direction of inter-hemispheric differences in SPSs over the sensorimotor regions apparent during the S2-S3 interval, under the VD condition, is similar to that observed in the SW condition. That is, for right response trials the SPS over the left sensorimotor area is more negative than that over the right area. The converse is true for left response trials, although the inter-hemispheric differences are much smaller in this case. Corresponding inter-hemispheric differences in SPSs did not occur in the S1-S2 interval of the VD condition, during which S was not preparing for an immediate overt motor response, but rather was attending to the S1 dot pattern preparatory to the discrimination required at S2. Figure 1 also shows superimposed, grand mean SPSs from $C_3$ and $C_4$ of 5 left-handed Ss during left and right response trials of the SW, GW and VD conditions. In general, these SPSs exhibit the same features as those for right-handed Ss. An exception is that the inter-hemispheric SPS differences during left response trials of SW and the S2-S3 interval of VD are smaller than those for right-handed Ss.

The data presented in figures 2–4 show the distribution of grand mean inter-hemispheric differences in SPSs over occipital ($O_1$-$O_2$), parietal ($P_3$-$P_4$), sensorimotor ($C_3$-$C_4$), and frontal ($F_3$-$F_4$) regions during the SW, GW, and VD conditions, respectively. In figures 2–4 upward deflections indicate that the left hemisphere was more negative than the right hemisphere at the indicated cortical regions. The inter-hemispheric SPS difference records for right and left response trials are superimposed to facilitate comparisons.

It will be noted in these figures that the difference curves for SPSs recorded over sensorimotor areas show the features observed in the superimposed records of figure 1 more clearly. During right response trials of

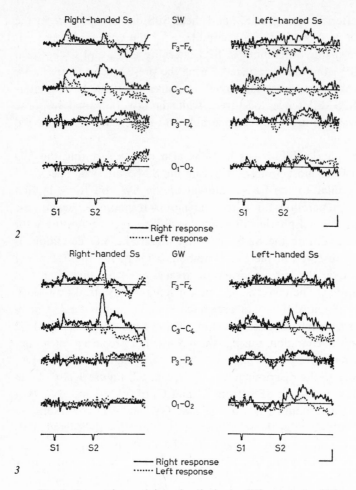

*Fig. 2.* Comparison of inter-hemispheric differences in SPSs recorded in the SW condition during right- and left-hand response trials. Records on the left are grand means of the separately averaged difference SPSs for 9 right-handed Ss. Records on the right are grand means of averaged difference SPSs for 5 left-handed Ss. Inter-hemispheric difference SPSs were obtained with transhemispheric, bipolar electrodes at $F_3$-$F_4$, $P_3$-$P_4$, and $O_1$-$O_2$ of the international 10–20 electrode system. Difference SPSs at C3-C4 were obtained by subtraction of SPSs recorded at $C_4$ from those recorded at $C_3$, with both $C_3$ and $C_4$ referenced to linked earlobe electrodes. Negativity is up at the left hemisphere relative to the right hemisphere electrode. Calibrations: 500 msec; 5 $\mu$V.

*Fig. 3.* Comparison of inter-hemispheric differences in SPSs recorded in the GW condition during right- and left-hand response trials (see legend of fig. 2 for details). Calibrations: 500 msec; 5 $\mu$V.

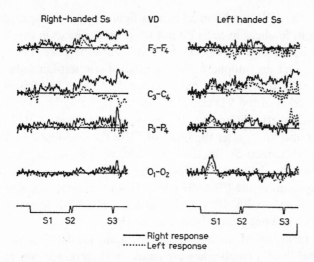

*Fig. 4.* Comparison of inter-hemispheric differences in SPSs recorded in the VD condition during right- and left-hand response trials (see legend of fig. 2 for details). Calibrations: 500 msec; 5 μV.

the SW condition, the left sensorimotor area is more negative than the right immediately after the S1 warning stimulus, and remains more negative throughout the warning interval and beyond the time of occurrence of the response to S2. The right sensorimotor area is more negative during left response trials, but not until about 500 msec before S2. Similar reciprocal, inter-hemispheric differences in SPS are not seen at cortical sites anterior or posterior to the sensorimotor area, except over the frontal area in left-handed subjects, but the differences there are appreciably smaller than at the sensorimotor region. A restriction of response-related, reciprocal, inter-hemispheric differences in SPSs to the sensorimotor region is also apparent during the motor interval of the VD condition shown in figure 4. Similar reciprocal differences can be seen in the frontal records of right-handed subjects in figure 4, but these differences are smaller than those over the sensorimotor area.

In the VD condition, shown in figure 4, no reciprocal, inter-hemispheric differences in SPSs are apparent during the S1-S2 interval at any of the electrode sites. After S2, when the subject knows which response to make, prepares for it and then makes it at S3, such reciprocal differences do occur, are similar to those seen in the SW condition, and are again largest over the sensorimotor area.

The data for the GW condition shown in figure 3 also indicate that inter-hemispheric differences in SPSs do not reflect differences in cerebral dominance. That is, the data do not exhibit consistent differences in inter-hemispheric SPSs that are uniquely related to right- or left-handedness. The same is generally true for inter-hemispheric differences in SPSs during the sensory interval of the VD condition seen in figure 4. The only appreciable interhemispheric differences in the sensory interval of the VD condition occur immediately after the onset of S1 in the occipital and parietal records of left-handed Ss. In those records, the left hemisphere is more negative than the right for a period of time that coincides with the late positive component of the EP to S1 onset. However, since the present study is concerned only with SPSs and inter-hemispheric differences in SPSs, EP amplitude will not be considered further here.

Quantitative measures of the average pre-S2 (and pre-S3) inter-hemispheric differences in SPS amplitude were made on the averages for each subject at each electrode site in the three conditions. A comparison of the means of these measures for left- and right-hand response trials are presented in figure 5A, B, C, and D for the SW and GW conditions, and for the sensory and motor intervals of the VD condition, respectively. Although inter-hemispheric differences in SPSs were smaller for left response trials in left-handed Ss than in right-handed Ss, the small number of left-handers precluded determination of statistical significance in this comparison. Since there were no other significant differences in inter-hemispheric SPSs, as is evident in figures 2–4, the mean values presented in figure 5 represent the combined data from right- and left-handed Ss.

In figure 5A, the amplitude of the inter-hemispheric SPS difference records during right and left response trials of the SW condition is clearly greater than zero only for the sensorimotor area. Results of Wilcoxon matched-pairs signed-ranks tests (one-tailed) for the SW condition confirmed that the inter-hemispheric differences were significant only at the sensorimotor region during both right ($p < 0.005$) and left ($p < 0.05$) response trials. In figure 5B, no appreciable, inter-hemispheric differences are seen at any electrode site in the GW condition for either right or left trials. A statistical comparison of these inter-hemispheric differences in the GW condition confirmed that there were no significant differences in SPS amplitude between left and right hemispheres when the subject could not prepare in advance for a unimanual motor response. As seen graphically in figure 5C, and confirmed statistically, no significant inter-hemispheric differences occurred during the sensory interval of the VD condi-

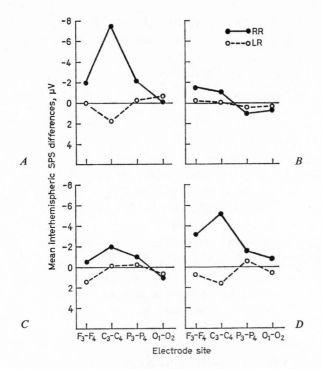

*Fig. 5.* Comparison of mean amplitudes of inter-hemispheric SPSs measured during trials requiring a right-hand response (solid line) with those measured during trials requiring a left-hand response (dashed line). Values in *A*, *B*, and *C* were means of the average amplitude over a 200-msec interval immediately prior to S2; those in *D* were measured prior to S3. Each data point represents the mean of 14 right- and left-handed Ss. *A* SW condition; *B* GW condition; *C* sensory phase (S1-S2 interval) of VD condition; *D* motor phase (S2-S3 interval) of VD condition.

tion when the subject was paying attention to a visual pattern. In contrast, figure 5D shows that during the motor interval of the VD condition, when the subject again was preparing to make a unimanual response, there were inter-hemispheric differences in SPSs; the left sensorimotor area was significantly more negative than the right when the response was to be a right response ($p < 0.01$, one-tail test), and vice versa when the response was a left response ($p < 0.05$, one-tail test). This finding replicates that made in the SW condition. The smaller SPS asymmetry over $C_3$-$C_4$ during left-response trials was not due to differences in RTs between left- and right-response trials. No significant differences between left- and right-hand RTs were found in the SW, GW, or VD conditions. Regardless of response hand, RTs in the SW condition were consistently shorter than in either the GW or VD conditions, which did not differ significantly from each other.

*In summary,* the foregoing data indicate that during warned preparation for a unilateral motor response, the SPS over sensorimotor cortex contralateral to the response is more negative than the SPS over the homologous, ipsilateral sensorimotor cortex. This reciprocal relationship between unimanual motor preparation and maximum SPS amplitude at the contralateral hemisphere does not occur in frontal, parietal or occipital cortical regions. Nor does it occur during preparation for a visual discrimination in the absence of unimanual motor readiness. Only when the *S* is allowed to prepare in advance either a right- or a left-hand response, does the inter-hemispheric asymmetry over the sensorimotor area become apparent. When the *S* prepares a left-hand response, the right sensorimotor region shows a more negative SPS than does the left, while when the *S* prepares a right-hand response, the left sensorimotor area is more negative than the right. The bilateral SPS asymmetry appears to be smaller for left response preparation, especially in left-handed *S*s.

### III. Midline SPSs and Motor vs. Sensory Task Requirements

The behavioral task typically used to elicit a vertex-CNV is the warned RT task or the paradigm S1-S2-R. The anterior-posterior scalp distribution of negative SPSs during the simple warned RT task exhibits a vertex maximum. The posterior potential gradient is steeper than the anterior, so that the SPS is generally smaller at the occiput than at the frontal pole [COHEN, 1969]. Variations in the behavioral task may be associated with different topographical distributions. For example, in a forewarned shock avoidance task, the site of maximum SPS amplitude appeared to shift toward more frontal regions [CANT and BICKFORD, 1967]. A decrease in the posterior potential gradient was noted during a difficult forewarned visual recognition task [COHEN, 1973], while the anterior gradient changed appreciably during an auditory discrimination task [JARVILEHTO and FRUHSTORFER, 1970]. The task-dependent changes in SPS topography are related to differences in the behavioral requirements of the tasks and to the presumed accompanying interplay of multiple intracortical SPS generators.

The results of the foregoing results in humans, which suggest the task-dependent modulation of multiple SPS generators, are not surprising in view of the findings on SPSs in animal studies. For example, in acute cat preparations it has been shown that repetitive electrical stimulation of non-specific, midline reticular formation or midline thalamic nuclei elicits SPSs of widespread cortical distribution, while stimulation of lateral thalamic nuclei elicits SPSs that are localized to the cortical projection area of the nuclei [ARDUINI et al., 1957; BROOKHART et al., 1958]. In chronic preparations, variations in topographical distribution of cortical SPSs have been associated with behavioral changes over time in a given experimental situation [BORDA, 1970; CHIORINI, 1969], with differing behavioral requirements within an experimental task [STAMM and ROSEN, 1969] and with different behavioral tasks [DONCHIN et al., 1971].

In the present study a set of sensory and motor tasks were selected to examine further the relationship between the midline scalp distribution of SPSs and specific task requirements. In particular, we examined the following hypotheses: (1) In a simple warned RT task, the midline distribution of SPSs should exhibit maximum negativity over central regions and a steeper posterior than anterior potential gradient. (2) During a disjunctive RT task with visual stimulation, in which there is a mixture of response and sensory preparatory sets, an SPS distribution similar to that in (1) was expected, but with a relative enhancement of posterior negativity. (3) In a visual discrimination task, scalp SPS distribution was expected to depend on the immediate requirements of the task. During preparation for the visual discrimination, in the absence of response preparation, greater involvement of posterior areas was expected. In the same temporal sequence of events, but during preparation for task related motor output, the distribution of negative SPSs was expected to be centrally dominant.

### Method

Nine undergraduates fulfilling course requirements served as subjects in one 2-hour experimental session. Recording procedures were the same as those described in part II, except that electrodes were placed along the midline over prefrontal (Fpz), frontal (Fz), central (Cz), parietal (Pz), and occipital (Oz) areas and referenced to linked earlobe electrodes. Vertical EOG was again monitored. The three experimental conditions used in the previous experiment were again presented to each S with the order counterbalanced across Ss. The conditions were the SW, GW, and VD conditions. The SW conditions provided a test of hypothesis 1, the GW a test of hypothesis 2, and the VD condition a test of hypothesis 3. In addition, a fourth condition, the visual control (VC) condition, was introduced to serve as a control for the VD task. In VC the S1, S2 and S3 stimuli were identical to those in the VD condition, but S was instructed only to make a right-hand key press to S3 regardless of the stimulus change at S2. The VC condition provided a control for the mere presentation of the visual patterns at S1 and S2. In all 4 conditions left- and right-hand response trials were averaged together.

## Results

The left side of figure 6 represents records which show the grand means of the averages from each of the 9 Ss for both the SW and GW conditions. The means of the amplitude measures for the 9 Ss constitute the data points plotted on the right side of figure 6. It will be noted that the Oz, Pz, Cz, and Fz electrode locations all showed a negative SPS, whereas the Fpz site showed a slight positive SPS. A Friedman two-way (subjects × electrode site) analysis of variance [SIEGEL, 1956] showed that the amplitudes at the various electrodes were significantly different under both the SW and GW conditions. Wilcoxon matched-pairs signed-ranks tests were made between SPSs from adjacent electrode sites, and showed that the SPS at Cz was significantly more negative than SPSs at other cortical sites. Also, there was a significant decreasing (less negative) potential gradient anteriorly and posteriorly from Cz in both the SW and GW conditions. The SPS amplitudes at corresponding sites under the two conditions were not significantly different.

Figure 7A shows that in the VD condition there was a negative-going shift during the attentive observation of the dot pattern exhibited between S1 and S2 at electrode sites Oz, Pz, and Cz. Such a negative-going shift did not occur at Fz or Fpz, where instead there were positive SPSs. During the motor preparatory interval between S2 and S3, there were negative SPS at Oz, Pz, and Cz, with the greatest amplitude exhibited at Cz and decreasing gradients both anteriorly and posteriorly. The Fpz site showed a slight positive SPS. These results during the motor preparatory phase of the VD task are similar to those just reported for the SW and GW conditions of the preceding motor tasks (SW and GW). In contrast, figure 7A also shows that during the VC condition, smaller SPS occurred at all electrode sites, although the direction of the shifts was similar to those in the VD condition.

Figures 7B and 7C show the quantitative values for the S1-S2 and the S2-S3 phases of the VD and VC tasks, respectively. In the VD-M and VC-M (motor preparatory intervals between S2 and S3) phases of the sensory tasks, Cz shows the largest amplitude negative SPS with decreasing gradients anteriorly and posteriorly. A Friedman analysis of variance showed that SPS amplitudes at the various electrode sites were signifi-

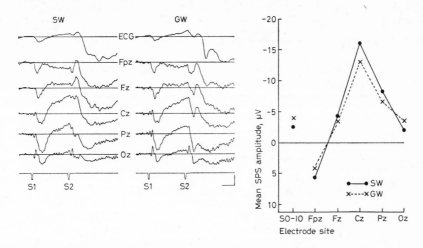

*Fig. 6.* Left: Longitudinal distribution of grand means of averaged SPSs for 9 Ss under the SW and GW conditions. In this and all subsequent figures, electrode sites Oz, Pz, Cz, Fz, and Fpz represent midline occipital, parietal, central, frontal, and prefrontal locations of international 10–20 electrode system, respectively; each electrode is referenced to linked earlobe leads. EOG = Vertical electro-oculogram recorded between superior (SO) and inferior orbital (IO) electrodes. Straight line through each graph is the pre-S1 baseline level of activity. Negativity upward at each scalp electrode site and at superior orbital electrode of the EOG. Calibrations: 500 msec; 10 μV. Right: Anterior-posterior distribution of pre-S2 SPS amplitudes measured in the SW and GW conditions. Each data point represents the mean of the separately measured average records of 9 Ss.

cantly different under both the VD-M and VC-M phases. Wilcoxon tests showed that the Cz region was significantly more negative than areas anterior and posterior. SPSs at Cz, Pz, and Oz were significantly more negative in the VD condition as compared to VC for both the S1-S2 and S2-S3 intervals.

With respect to the changes in SPSs which occurred during the S1-S2 phase of the VD-S and VC-S conditions, it is to be noted that a similar pattern of shift occurred in both conditions. An analysis of variance showed that SPS amplitudes were significantly different between adjacent electrode sites in both the VD and VC conditions. Individual comparisons between sites showed that in the VD-S condition, SPSs at Cz and Oz were significantly more negative than SPSs at adjacent sites, but did not differ from each other, in contrast with the results for VD-M. In the VD-S condition, the only significant difference was greater negativity at Oz com-

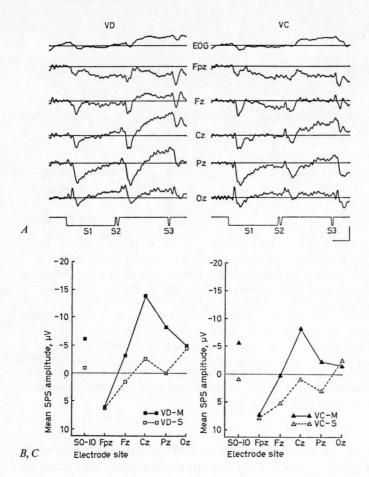

*Fig. 7.* Topographical distributions of averaged SPSs for 9 *S*s under the VD and VC conditions. *A* Midsagittal distribution of grand mean SPSs in VD and VC. Calibration: 500 msec; 10 μV. *B* Anterior-posterior distribution of pre-S2 (VD-S) and pre-S3 (VD-M) amplitudes measured in the VD condition. *C* Anterior-posterior distribution of pre-S2 (VC-s) and pre-S3 (VC-M) amplitudes measured in the VC condition. Each data point in *B* and *C* represents the means of the separately measured averaged SPSs of 9 *S*s at the indicated electrode site.

pared with Pz. Comparisons between VD-S and VC-S showed that only SPSs at Cz, Pz and Oz were significantly more negative in the VD-S condition.

In contrasting VD-M and VD-S (S2-S3 vs. S1-S2 phases) in figure 7, it will be noted that the Cz location has a much larger negative SPS in VD-M, thus associating a larger change in the SPS of the Cz area with the motor preparatory phase of the task. The same finding was true for the VC-M and VC-S phases, despite the overall smaller amplitude of SPSs during the VC task. It is also important to note that the increase in SPS amplitude at Cz from the sensory to motor phases of both VD and VC was not paralleled by the SPS at Oz or at Fpz. SPS amplitude at Oz was not significantly different from the amplitude at Cz during the sensory phase and did not follow the increase at Cz during the motor phase. Thus, SPSs at Oz and Cz were dissociated between the sensory and motor phases of the VD and VC conditions. This was also the case for SPSs at Fpz and Cz.

The mean RTs across the 9 Ss in the SW, GW, VD, and VC conditions were 254, 413, 435, and 409 msec, respectively. The RTs in SW were significantly shorter than in the other three conditions, which did not differ significantly in RT from each other. A comparison between SPS amplitude and RT showed that the two measures were not related across conditions. Although there were no significant differences between SPS amplitudes at Cz in the SW and GW, and VD-M conditions, RTs were significantly shorter in SW than in GW or VD. Discrimination performance in VD was above 90% correct for all subjects, so that no comparisons could be made among correct and incorrect trials and SPS amplitude.

*In summary,* we confirmed the typical finding of a centrally dominant SPS distribution during preparation for motor responses, but failed to confirm the nature of the anterior and posterior potential gradients. In fact, the data were directly opposite to previous findings, exhibiting instead steeper anterior than posterior gradients of negativity. The expected enhancement of posterior negativity during a disjunctive RT task with visual stimuli was also not obtained. However, we did find a dissociation between occipital and central SPSs during the sensory and motor phases of a visual discrimination task. The fact that a similar dissociation of SPSs at Cz and Oz was noted in the control task (VC), suggests that preparation for the VD was not critical for the dissociation. An unexpected dissociation between SPSs at Fpz and Cz was also found.

## IV. Midline SPSs and Modality of Sensory Stimulation

In the study described above, we found midline SPS distributions in warned RT tasks that differed in the anterior and posterior extent of the negative SPS gradient from that obtained in other investigations. Our study also differed methodologically from earlier studies in our exclusive use of visual stimuli for S1, S2, S3, and RT feedback. It is possible that this unimodal stimulation procedure, as opposed to the typical bimodal paradigm employed in most CNV studies, was instrumental in producing the distributions we found.

In order to examine systematically the effect of modality on SPS distribution, we presented motor and sensory tasks that differed only in the modality of S1, S2, S3, and feedback. Task behavioral requirements were identical, while modality of stimulation was either solely auditory or visual. In addition, auditory and visual trials of a given experimental task were randomly intermixed to preclude the formation of differential tonic stimulus or response sets. Performance, in the form of reaction times or discrimination errors, was also monitored and provided an independent measure of the extent to which task requirements were being met in the trials for each modality.

### Method

Five Ss were run in two experimental situations. The first was a warned RT task in which two conditions were randomly intermixed. In the visual motor (VM) condition, both S1 and S2 were 50-msec displays of a dot pattern, while in the auditory motor (AM) condition, S1 and S2 were 50-msec, 1,000-Hz tone pips. The ISI was 1.5 sec, and identical finger responses to S2 were required in AM and VM. Reaction time feedback was presented visually in VM, while in AM feedback was presented in the auditory mode (i.e. verbally).

The second experimental situation involved presentation of two randomly intermixed sensory discrimination tasks. In the VD condition, 50-msec displays of a dot pattern were presented at S1 and S2. The S was instructed to discriminate in which direction the pattern at S2 was shifted relative to a standard position at S1. In the auditory discrimination (AD) condition, S1 and S2 were 50-msec tone pips and the S was instructed to discriminate the direction of pitch change of the tone at S2 relative to a standard 1,000-Hz tone at S1. In both VD and AD the S1-S2 and S2-S3 ISIs were each 1.5 sec. The word REPORT was presented visually at S3 and instructed S to press right- or left-hand switches in order to report the results of the discrimination.

The recording procedures, midline electrode sites, and data analyses were identical to those described for the previous experiment.

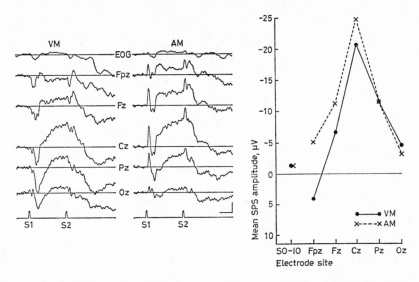

*Fig. 8.* Left: Midsagittal distribution of grand means of averaged SPSs for 5 Ss under the VM and AM conditions. Calibrations: 500 msec; 10 μV; negativity up. Right: Anterior-posterior distribution of pre-S2, mean amplitudes measured in the VM and AM conditions. Each data point represents the means of the separately measured records of 5 *Ss*.

## Results

The left side of figure 8 shows grand mean SPS curves for the 5 Ss during the VM and AM conditions, while on the right side, each data point of the plots represents the mean of the separately measured, pre-S2, average amplitudes for the same Ss at each electrode site. It will be noted that mean SPS amplitudes over Cz, Fz, and Fpz during AM are more negative than the corresponding amplitudes during the VM task. The reverse is true for SPS amplitude at Oz. To determine whether the observed differences in SPS distribution were consistent across subjects, ratios of SPS amplitude at Fpz, Fz, Pz, and Oz relative to the amplitude at Cz were calculated for each subject in AM and VM. The Fpz:Cz ratios were larger in AM than in VM for all five subjects. The reverse was true for the Oz:Cz ratios in four of the five subjects. The same four out of five subjects showed larger Fz:Cz and Pz:Cz ratios in AM than in VM. Thus, relative to SPS amplitude at Cz, SPS amplitudes at Fpz, Fz, and Pz were larger with auditory stimulation than with visual, while the occipital SPS was larger with visual stimulation than with auditory. These differences in

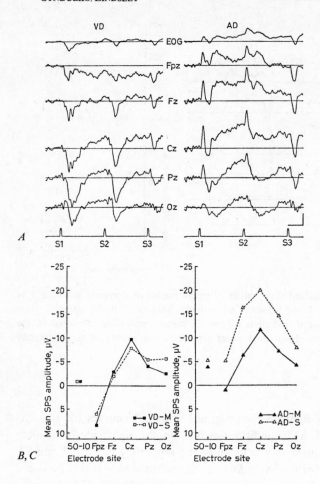

*Fig. 9.* Topographical distributions of the means of averaged SPSs for 5 Ss under the VD and AD conditions. *A* Midline distribution of grand mean SPSs in VD and VC. Calibration: 500 msec; 10 $\mu$V. *B* Anterior-posterior distribution of pre-S2 (VD-S) and pre-S3 (VD-M) SPS amplitudes measured in the VD condition. *C* Anterior-posterior distribution of pre-S2 (AD-S) and pre-S3 (AD-M) SPS amplitudes in the AD condition. Each data point in B and C represents the means of the separately measured, averaged SPSs of 5 Ss at the indicated electrode site.

relative SPS distribution under conditions of auditory and visual stimulation were not due to differences in general level of arousal between the AM and VM tasks, since trials of the two tasks were randomly intermixed. Rather, the differences in SPS distribution between AM and VM appear to be related to differences in the modality of stimulation used in the two tasks. It should be noted that four out of five $S$s showed shorter RTs in AM ($\bar{X} = 253$ msec) than in VM ($\bar{X} = 278$ msec). The RT difference suggests that auditory stimulation may be phasically more arousing or alerting than visual stimulation.

One additional feature to note in the grand mean curves shown in figure 8 is the shape of the SPSs over Fpz in VM, but particularly in AM. In both conditions, the SPS at Fpz reaches an initial negative maximum about 500–600 msec after S1 and after S2. The short latency SPS decreases in amplitude to a lower level throughout the remainder of the S1-S2 interval, while after S2 it quickly returns to baseline. A similar short latency, negative SPS occurs at Fz, but it is quickly followed by the slowly rising negative SPS characteristic of more central areas during the S1-S2 interval, particularly at Cz. The short latency SPS is almost totally absent at Pz and Oz. The distribution of the short latency SPS is similar to that described for SPS during auditory discrimination tasks in the absence of motor preparation [JARVILEHTO and FRUHSTORFER, 1970]. However, it seems clear that in the AM and VM tasks, the short latency, frontally dominant SPS is not related to the 'uncertainty' of a discrimination task as proposed by JARVILEHTO and FRUHSTORFER [1970].

Grand mean SPSs for the VD and AD conditions are presented in figure 9A. The means of the separately measured (for each $S$) average amplitudes for the pre-S2 (VD-S and AD-S) and pre-S3 (VD-M and AD-M) intervals are shown in figure 9B and C, respectively. During the S1-S2 interval of VD, negative SPSs were most prominent at Cz, Pz, and Oz; the SPS at Fpz was positive in polarity. During the S2-S3, SPSs were largest at Fz, Cz, and Pz. The Cz site exhibited the largest negative amplitudes during both the S1-S2 and S2-S3 intervals, and did not show a consistent change in amplitude between the two intervals. Likewise, SPS amplitudes at Fpz, Fz, and Pz were not consistently different between the S1-S2 and S2–S3 intervals. In contrast, SPSs at Oz were larger (more negative) during preparation for the visual discrimination (S1-S2 interval) than during motor response preparation (S2-S3 interval) for four out of five $S$s. The data confirm the independence of SPSs over central and occipital regions during the sensory and motor phases of a visual discrimination task.

In both the S1-S2 and S2-S3 intervals of the AD conditions, maximum negative SPSs occurred at Cz and decreased monotonically both anteriorly and posteriorly. A comparison of the pre-S2 (AD-S) and pre-S3 (AD-M) mean amplitudes for AD (fig. 9C) showed that SPSs were larger at all electrode sites during the S1-S2 interval. The differences were most consistent at Cz and Fz, although no clear dissociations among SPSs at different electrode sites were found.

A comparison of the amplitude plots for VD-S and AD-S (fig. 9B and C, respectively) shows that the absolute magnitudes of SPSs at all sites in AD-S are greater than those in VD-S. However, when ratios were calculated for SPS amplitude at Oz, Pz, Fz, and Fpz relative to the amplitude at Cz, a different picture emerged. Four of the five Ss showed larger Oz:Cz ratios for VD-S than for AD-S. The same four Ss showed larger Fpz:Cz and Fz:Cz ratios for AD-S than for VD-S. Thus, when relative amplitude differences were considered, SPS amplitudes were enhanced at Oz during visual attentiveness, and were enhanced at Fpz and Fz during auditory attentiveness.

The distribution of SPSs during the motor preparatory interval (S2-S3) of the AD condition was similar to that during the same interval of the VD condition. The most consistent difference between the VD and AD conditions for the S2-S3 interval was the size of the positive SPS at Fpz; a large, consistently positive SPS occurred in VD, while a considerably smaller, and less consistently positive SPS occurred in AD. A short latency, negative SPS at Fpz, which is similar to that noted above in the VM and AM conditions, was again evident after S1 and S2 in the AD condition (fig. 9A). As in the VM and AM conditions, the short latency SPS was independent of the slower rising, negative SPS that peaks at S2 and exhibits maximum amplitude over central regions. The short latency SPS was not evident during the VD condition.

*In summary,* modality effects were found for the distribution of SPSs during RT and sensory discrimination tasks. SPSs were relatively enhanced over the occipital region when visual stimulation was employed, while the reverse was true for SPSs over frontal regions during auditory stimulation.

## V. SPSs and Voluntary Eye Movements

Previous studies have demonstrated that SPSs originating at the eyes and accompanying downward eye movements can seriously distort recordings of scalp SPSs made at the vertex and over frontal regions [HILL-YARD and GALAMBOS, 1969; STRAUMANIS *et al.*, 1969; WASMAN *et al.*, 1970]. To minimize the effects of eye movement artifact on SPSs, a fixation point was employed in the present experiments. However, since the contamination of scalp SPS by ocular potentials may occur in some subjects even when fixated [WASMAN *et al.*, 1970], simultaneous recordings of the vertical EOG were made during all experimental procedures. The horizontal EOG was not monitored because pilot studies showed that use of a linked-earlobe reference for SPS recordings precluded their contamination by horizontal eye movements.

In order to provide a standard of comparison by which to distinguish artifactually produced potential gradients from those that might accompany experimental manipulations, recordings of midline potential gradients accompanying voluntary eye movements were made in two subjects.

To facilitate event-locked averaging of potentials accompanying voluntary eye movements, a three stimulus paradigm was used in which S1, S2, and S3 were visual stimuli separated by onset-to-onset ISIs of 1.5 sec. Three fixation points were provided during each run of 32 trials (i.e. presentations of S1, S2, and S3). The standard point was located at the center of the CRT. Fixation points were also positioned equal distances directly above and below the standard point. The distance between adjacent points was varied between runs to permit eye displacements of 1.25 and 2.5° of visual angle in *S* GW, and 5 and 10° in *S* DS. The *S* was instructed to fixate the center point between trials. At S1, *S* quickly moved his eyes to the upward fixation point and fixated it until S2. At S2, *S* moved his eyes rapidly downward to the lower fixation point and fixated it until S3, whereupon he again fixated the center point.

Averages at each electrode were taken separately over trials of a given displacement. Figure 10 (left side) shows the distribution of averaged potentials at the eye (vertical EOG) and over the head during 1.25, 2.5, 5, and 10° upward (S1-S2 interval) and downward (S2-S3 interval) eye displacements. Figure 10 (right side) presents plots of the longitudinal distribution of potentials measured during downward eye displacements of 10, 5, 2.5, and 1.5°. Figure 10 shows that the magnitude of the EOG (relative to pre-S1 baseline and center fixation) is positively related to the extent of angular displacement of the eyes; the greater the displacement, the larger the EOG (note difference in calibrations between the records).

The size of scalp SPSs simultaneously recorded at midline electrodes also was related to the extent of ocular displacement, particularly for

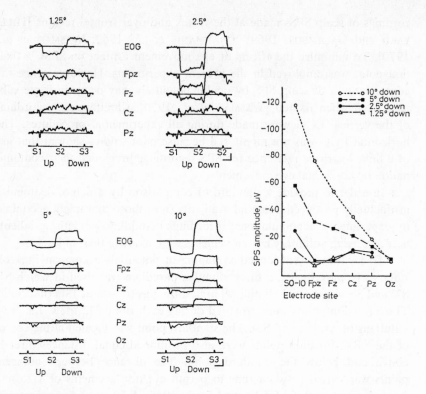

*Fig. 10.* Left: Midsagittal distribution of average SPSs accompanying maintained, voluntary upward (S1-S2 interval) and downward (S2-S3 interval) displacements of the eye. Left upper: Subject GW – 1.25 and 2.5° eye movement excursions. Left lower: Subject DS = 5 and 10° excursions. Calibration: 500 msec; 10 μV (upper), 40 μV (lower); negativity at active electrode is up. Right: Anterior-posterior distribution of SPS amplitude measures during 1.25, 2.5, 5, and 10° downward eye movements. Each data point represents the average amplitude over a 200-msec epoch prior to S3. Measures were made on curves shown at the left.

SPSs over frontal regions. For the 5 and 10° movements, there was a monotonically decreasing gradient of potentials (except at Oz) with maximum amplitudes at Fpz. The change in potential at Cz between the downward 5 and 10° movements was 11 μV, which corresponds to a 58-μV change in the EOG; the concurrent potential change at Fpz was 43 μV. The attenuation factor at Cz is about 5:1, while that at Fpz is about 0.8:1 for this *S*.

The effects on scalp SPSs of ocular potentials accompanying the 1.25 and 2.5° eye movements were considerably less than for the 5 and 10° movements, especially for central and posterior sites. In spite of a 15-$\mu$V difference in EOG amplitude for downward eye displacements between the 2.5 and 1.25° movements, the change in potential at Cz that might be related to the EOG change was 1 $\mu$V, while that at Fpz was only 3 $\mu$V. The very rapid decrease in EOG artifact with increasing distance from the eye suggests an exponential decay.

*In summary*, we may conclude that the effect on scalp recorded SPSs of EOG artifact less than 20 $\mu$V in amplitude appears to be minimal, especially for electrode sites posterior to Fz. The main effect of EOG artifact for downward eye movements is to cause a frontally dominant, negative potential gradient. Therefore, the SPS distributions obtained on the three experiments described above can be clearly distinguished from SPSs resulting from vertical ocular displacements. It is interesting to note in figure 10 that the anterior-posterior midline potential gradient during preparation for small eye movements was similar to that obtained during the motor preparatory intervals of the reaction-time tasks, i.e. both showed maximum negativity at Cz with decreasing amplitudes posteriorly and anteriorly.

## VI. Discussion

The primary goal of these experiments was to investigate the topographical distribution of SPSs in tasks which emphasized either motor readiness or sensory attentiveness. It was felt that knowledge of the topographical distribution of scalp recorded SPSs under different behavioral conditions could lead to a clearer understanding of the functional significance of SPSs.

We have observed that in all conditions (SW, GW, AM, VM, VD-M, AD-M, VC-M) during which Ss prepared for a motor response, there was a characteristic anterior-posterior, midline distribution of negative SPSs during the preparatory interval. The maximum negative SPS always occurred over the central or motor regions (Cz), and there was a monotonically decreasing gradient of negative potentials both anteriorly and posteriorly. The consistency of this finding across conditions and subjects was striking. The centrally dominant distribution occurred in simple, warned reaction time tasks (SW, VM, and AM conditions), in a disjunctive reaction time task (GW), and during preparation for non-imperative, but task-related, motor output (VD-M and AD-M). The primary feature of the distribution, i.e. a central SPS maximum with decreasing gradients anteriorly and posteriorly, also appeared to be independent of stimulus modality.

The focus of maximum negativity of SPSs recorded along the midline during motor preparation was over cortical motor areas. The central focus and the relationship of the central SPSs to motor preparation suggests that the SPSs are relatively localized electrocortical changes which underlie motor preparation and readiness to respond. This view is strongly supported by the results of the lateral distribution study, which examined the relationship between unimanual response preparation and the hemispheric focus of SPSs. It was shown that during preparation for a unimanual response, as in the SW and VD-M conditions, the SPS over the sensorimotor region contralateral to the intended response was more negative than the SPS over the homologous ipsilateral area. Thus, the electrocortical change with unimanual motor preparation was even more localized, i.e. to the sensorimotor area of one hemisphere. Laterality effects did not occur or were considerably attenuated in frontal, parietal, and occipital regions. In addition, the hemispheric asymmetry in SPS amplitude was not evident during bimanual response preparation (GW condition), nor during the attentive observation of visual input in the absence of unimanual response preparation (VD-S condition). The laterality effect was observed in both right- and left-handed Ss and for both right- and left-hand responses, although some differences were noted in left-handed Ss and for left-hand responses (see below).

Another finding generally consistent with a motor readiness, or a motor set, interpretation of the functional significance of central SPSs was the distribution of SPSs during the sensory and motor intervals of the discrimination tasks. Central SPSs were recorded in the absence of immediate motor preparation during the sensory intervals of the discrimination tasks (VD-S and AD-S). It might be expected that the amplitude of central SPSs would be less during the sensory interval than during the motor interval, if the central SPSs are in fact more closely related to motor preparation. This was found to be true in condition VD, where the difference in central SPS amplitudes between the sensory and motor preparatory intervals was highly significant. The primary difference in the midline longitudinal potential gradient between the two intervals reflected a relative absence of central SPSs during the sensory interval (VD-S), and the subsequent development of SPSs during the motor interval (VD-M). SPS amplitude over the visual cortex did not show a similar pattern of development, thus indicating that the absence of central SPS in the sensory interval was not the result of a generalized deficiency of SPS development. Rather, the results for midline topogaphical distribution in the VD condition support the view that the temporal development of central, negative, SPSs is associated with motor preparatory processes.

The results of the VD and AD tasks were not as consistent. In the VD condition of the modality study, the mean SPS amplitudes over central areas were similar during the sensory and motor intervals, while in the AD condition mean SPSs were larger during the sensory interval. The larger central SPSs under conditions of auditory stimulation may reflect the presence of central SPSs specifically related to auditory stimulation (see below). The lack of a mean difference in SPS amplitude between the sensory and motor intervals of the visual task may reflect the idiosyncratic reactions of the Ss to the contrived separation of sensory and motor preparatory phases.

Although the results thus far discussed are generally consistent with the view that central SPSs are related to motor preparatory processes, the nature of the relationship is unclear. For example, although SPS amplitude over the sensorimotor cortex contralateral to a unimanual response was greater than that over ipsilateral cortex, the absolute magnitude of the ipsilateral SPS was substantial. The inter-hemispheric differences in SPS amplitudes appear to reflect localized electrocortical changes accompanying cortical processes specifically related to the intended response. However, the size of the ipsilateral sensorimotor SPS suggests concurrent, more generalized (bilateral) preparatory activity [cf. DEECKE and KORNHUBER, this volume]. Furthermore, since the lateral asymmetry in SPS amplitude persists for a few hundred milliseconds after completion of the response, the central SPSs may be related more to changes in somatic input than to response preparation *per se* [cf. GERBRANDT *et al.*, 1973]. The central SPSs during motor preparation may consist of separate SPSs that are related to both generalized motor set and specific response preparation. The present data do not indicate whether the SPSs primarily reflect excitatory or inhibitory processes, e.g. readiness to respond, or the temporary withholding or restraint of responses.

In most other studies, the central SPSs discussed above are called the CNV, and in the discussion that follows the term CNV will be restricted to SPSs at the vertex or central region. The present results are generally consistent with those of most other studies in which the midsagittal distribution of SPSs has been recorded in humans during a foreperiod reaction time task [CANT and BICKFORD, 1967; COHEN, 1969; JARVILEHTO and FRUHSTORFER, 1970; WALTER, 1967]. These studies all showed that maximum negative amplitude occurred at Cz during motor preparation. The results of the earlier distribution studies differ from those of this study in the relative extents of the potential gradients anterior and posterior to Cz. We find that the relative steepness of the anterior and posterior gradients depends on the stimulus modality used for S1 and S2. Steeper anterior than posterior gradients were obtained with visual stimulation, while the reverse was true for auditory stimulation. Steep anterior gradients, with occasional prefrontal positivity, were obtained in a study of SPS distributions during a warned reaction time task with visual stimulation [JARVILEHTO and FRUHSTORFER, 1970]. Because full details of the other studies cited above have not been published [CANT and BICKFORD, 1967; COHEN, 1969; WALTER, 1967], it is difficult to evaluate the modality of stimuli used and the artifact control procedures (for EOG artifact) employed.

The longitudinal distributions obtained in the present study during warned reaction time tasks with visual stimulation are similar to the distribution of the slow negative component of SPSs preceding uncued, voluntary movements [DEECKE et al., 1969; GERBRANDT et al., 1973; JARVILEHTO and FRUHSTORFER, 1970; VAUGHAN et al., 1968]. In the latter studies, the distribution of potentials immediately preceding voluntary muscle contractions also showed frontal pole positivity and a maximum negative amplitude over motor areas. The similarity in distribution and behavioral correlates between the 'readiness potential' on the one hand and the CNV during warned reaction time tasks on the other supports the view that the two types of SPSs reflect common physiological mechanisms.

The readiness potential, or the early negative SPS preceding voluntary, uncued movements, has an asymmetrical lateral distribution, such that the amplitude over motor cortex contralateral to the response is larger than that over ipsilateral motor cortex [DEECKE et al., 1973; GERBRANDT et al., 1973; GILDEN et al., 1966; McADAM and SEALES, 1969; VAUGHAN et al., 1968]. An asymmetrical distribution of SPSs was also found during warned unimanual motor preparation in the present study. Another recent study of SPS distribution during warned reaction time tasks also showed an asymmetrical distribution of potentials similar to the one obtained here [OTTO and LEIFER, 1973]. Two other studies failed to show bilateral asymmetry over motor areas [Low *et al.*, 1966; Cohen, 1969].

The discrepancy in the nature of the lateral distribution of SPS during warned RT tasks is puzzling and requires comment. We propose that the following variables are critically relevant for demonstrating bilateral asymmetries during externally cued preparation for motor output:

1) Explicit instructions and practice trials that emphasize differential preparation of left versus right limb responses: The typical RT paradigm in which lateral asymmetries were investigated in earlier studies [Cohen, 1969; Low *et al.*, 1966] involved emphasis on only one response side, e.g. right-hand responses. Presumably no explicit instructions were given about preparation of the non-responding limb, thus allowing considerable 'subject option' regarding preparation of that limb; for a discussion of the need for explicit instructions in experimental design, see Sutton [1969]. It should be noted that we found a bilaterally symmetrical distribution of SPSs during explicitly instructed, bimanual response preparation.

2) Random intermixture of left- and right-hand response trials: This random intermixture prevents the adoption of possible unimanual response sets that might be associated with differential tonic shifts in the resting EEG potential level over the two hemispheres.

3) Response limb: The bilateral SPS asymmetries over sensorimotor cortex were smaller during preparation for left finger response as compared to preparation for right finger responses. The effect of response hand on the size of the SPS asymmetry may be related to the finding that the left and right sensorimotor hemispheres exhibit fundamentally different organizational plans [Semmes, 1968]. Right limb functions were found to be more focally represented in the left hemisphere than left limb functions are represented in the right hemisphere. The left hemisphere also appears to exert more focal ipsilateral control than does the right hemisphere. In the warned RT task, the left sensorimotor region may be more active during preparation for left finger responses than is the right sensorimotor region during preparation for right finger responses. Our data suggest that the relative amplitude of negative SPSs over the two hemispheres during a warned RT task may provide a direct measure of the relative functional involvement of the hemispheres in motor preparatory activity. Similar suggestions have been made for SPSs preceding uncued, distal muscle contractions [Vaughan *et al.*, 1968], and for SPSs preceding speech [McAdam and Whitaker, 1971; cf. this series, vol. 3].

4) Hand preference: Left-handed *S*s showed smaller bilateral asym-

metries during left-response preparation than did right-handed Ss. This finding is similar to that reported for bilateral asymmetries of the early negative SPS preceding uncued hand movements [DEECKE et al., 1973; KUTAS and DONCHIN, this volume]. In turn, both of these findings probably reflect reported differences in cerebral organization between right- and left-handed Ss; left-handed Ss exhibit less intra- and inter-hemispheric focalization of a variety of functions [HÉCAEN and AJURIAGUERRA, 1964]. If the findings are confirmed and extended, determination of the degree of asymmetry of SPSs preceding either cued or uncued motor responses could provide the basis for diagnostic tests of the extent of cerebral lateralization of motor function, and of the intra- and inter-hemispheric focalization of sensorimotor functions.

TECCE [1972] recently proposed a dual-process model to explain certain CNV findings. In this model, both general arousal and selective attention are viewed as principal determinants of CNV amplitude. The present data support the view that central SPSs, here equated with the CNV, are primarily related to motor preparatory processes of both a general and specific character. The data are consonant with TECCE's model, if motor attention is substituted for sensory attention (to S2). Further support for this view is found in reviewing the effects of competing tasks on CNV amplitude in a warned RT task. In general, decreased CNV amplitudes were found when a competing *cognitive* task is superimposed on the RT task [MCCALLUM and WALTER, 1968; TECCE and SCHEFF, 1969]. In contrast, LOW and MCSHERRY [1968] reported that superimposition of two different, foreperiod RT tasks resulted in CNV amplitude *larger* than that present in either task alone. The apparent discrepancy can be explained on the basis of the degree of response compatibility of the superimposed tasks. When the superimposed tasks involved different task stimuli, but compatible motor responses, CNV amplitude increased [LOW and MCSHERRY, 1968]. When the tasks involve different stimuli and very different responses, i.e. cognitive versus overt motor responses, CNV decreased [MCCALLUM and WALTER, 1968; TECCE and SCHEFF, 1969]. Thus, the amplitude of the CNV was related directly to preparation for, or attention to, motor output, rather than to attention to task relevant stimuli.

Thus far, topographical distributions in particular behavioral tasks have been related to a certain extent to the presumed functional significance of SPSs recorded during motor preparation. In this view, central SPSs recorded during motor preparation are presumed to reflect cortical

activity which underlies motor readiness or motor set, of either a generalized or specific character [DONALD and GOFF, 1973]. A number of investigators have shown that central SPSs may occur in the absence of an overt motor response when the subject is asked to prepare to do arithmetic
calculations [DONCHIN et al., 1972], to anticipate a confirmatory stimulus
[DONCHIN et al., 1972; PICTON and LOW, 1971], or to make some decision which would be reported at a later time [COHEN and WALTER, 1966].
These tasks were assumed to be 'non-motor' in character, and it has been
argued that the presence of central SPS during such tasks proves that the
central SPSs are not solely related to motor preparatory processes [CO-
HEN, 1969; DONCHIN et al., 1972]. It is not certain, however, that even
these operations are devoid of all motor elements, particularly of a generalized response readiness. In fact, it can be argued that because central
SPSs are so prominent during motor preparation, their occurrence during
behaviors not involving immediate, *overt* motor acts suggests that these
behaviors are also 'motor' in character. There is insufficient evidence to
decide between these two possibilities.

SPERRY [1952] has suggested that regardless of the manifest behavioral situation, the primary end-product of the brain is motor output. The
ubiquitous central SPS may be an electrocortical expression of the degree
of cortical involvement in preparation for all varieties of motor output,
both over and covert. Situations not involving specific, overt motor responses may nevertheless produce generalized effector readiness, receptor
orientation, and non-automatic postural adjustments, in addition to specific motor concomitants of mental processes.

An examination of the topographical distribution of SPSs during the
sensory discrimination tasks has provided evidence for the existence of
localized SPSs specifically related to stimulation of a particular modality.
In the visual discrimination tasks, SPSs over occipital, prefrontal and
central regions were shown to be unrelated or independent, and thus
suggestive of localized generators of SPSs. The occipital SPS is presumably related to preparation for the processing of visual input and appears
to be similar to localized SPSs over occipital regions recorded in animals
[KÖHLER and O'CONNELL, 1957; ROSEN, 1969].

The prefrontal, positive SPS was a consistent concomitant of visual
stimulation regardless of the requirements of the immediate task. The
positive SPS occurred in all conditions of the three experiments in which
visual stimulation was employed. The close association with visual input,
and the proximity of the Fpz electrode to the eye, suggests that the posi-

tive SPS at Fpz may be related to the c-wave of the electroretinogram. The c-wave is a long latency positive shift (corneal positivity with respect to the back of the eye) of extended duration that is optimally produced by high levels of illumination against a relatively dark background. However, positive SPSs over the frontal pole have been described in the absence of visual stimulation (see discussion of readiness potential above). In the auditory discrimination task, positive SPSs at Fpz were obtained in three Ss during the interval between an auditory stimulus (S2) and a visual stimulus (S3). Further research is needed to determine the extent of contribution of light evoked electro-ocular potentials to frontally recorded SPSs.

In the auditory tasks (AM and AD), SPSs over frontal and central regions were considerably more negative than during the corresponding visual tasks (VM and VD). In fact, the distribution of negative SPSs during the auditory tasks was similar to the distribution of the major negative component of the auditory evoked potential. It has been suggested that due to the orientation of the auditory cortex in man relative to the surface, potentials generated in auditory cortex should appear at maximum amplitude at or slightly anterior to the vertex [KÖHLER and WEGENER, 1955]. Thus, the enhanced negative SPSs over central and frontal areas obtained in this study during auditory tasks may reflect the influence of electrocortical changes specific to auditory input or the anticipation of auditory input. Although the differences reported were not significant, SPSs at the vertex during a warned reaction time task were found to be more negative with auditory stimulation than with visual [LOW *et al.*, 1966; REBERT and KNOTT, 1970], thus adding support to the current finding.

The general conclusion of this study is that the topographical distribution of SPSs is sensitive to both the motor and sensory requirements of tasks involving preparatory intervals. Within the limits imposed by the relatively widespread electrode arrays employed in this study, fairly sharp regional differentiations could be made, particularly for SPSs related to visual stimulation and to unimanual motor preparation. Overlapping and interaction of different potential distributions also occurred, as in the case of SPSs over central and frontal regions associated with auditory stimulation and motor readiness. General characteristics of the potential distributions are similar to some of those described in animal studies [SYNDULKO, 1972], and thus invite comparisons and possible deductions as to the physiological basis and functional significance of the SPSs and their accompanying behaviors.

## References

ARDUINI, A.; MANCIA, M., and MECHELSE, K.: Slow potential changes elicited in the cerebral cortex by sensory and reticular stimulation. Arch. ital. Biol. 95: 127–128 (1957).

BORDA, R. P.: The effect of altered drive states on the contingent negative variation (CNV) in rhesus monkeys. Electroenceph. clin. Neurophysiol. 29: 173–180 (1970).

BROOKHART, J. M.; ARDUINI, A.; MANCIA, M., and MORUZZI, G.: Thalamocortical relations as revealed by induced slow potential changes. J. Neurophysiol. 21: 499–525 (1958).

CANT, B. R. and BICKFORD, R. G.: The effect of motivation on the contingent negative variation (CNV). Electroenceph. clin. Neurophysiol. 23: 594 (1967).

CHIORINI, J. R.: Slow potential changes from cat cortex and classical aversive conditioning. Electroenceph. clin. Neurophysiol. 26: 399–405 (1969).

COHEN, J.: Very slow brain potentials relating to expectancy: the CNV; in DONCHIN and LINDSLEY Average evoked potentials. NASA SP-191, pp. 143–198 (US Government Printing Office, Washington 1969).

COHEN, J.: The CNV and visual recognition. Electroenceph. clin. Neurophysiol. Suppl. 33: 201–204 (1973).

COHEN, J. and WALTER, W. G.: The interaction of responses in the brain to semantic stimuli. Psychophysiology 2: 187–196 (1966).

DEECKE, L.; BECKER, W.; GROZINGER, B.; SCHEID, P., and KORNHUBER, H.: Human brain potentials preceding voluntary limb movements. Electroenceph. clin. Neurophysiol. Suppl. 33: 87–94 (1973).

DEECKE, L.; SCHEID, P., and KORNHUBER, H. A.: Distribution of readiness potential, pre-motion positivity, and motor potential of the human cerebral cortex preceding voluntary finger movements. Expl Brain Res. 7: 158–168 (1968).

DONALD, M. W. and GOFF, W. R.: Discussion on CNV and human behavior. Electroenceph. clin. Neurophysiol. Suppl. 33: 241–242 (1973).

DONCHIN, E.; GERBRANDT, L. A.; LEIFER, L., and TUCKER, L.: Is the contingent negative variation contingent on a motor response? Psychophysiology 9: 178–188 (1972).

DONCHIN, E.; OTTO, D.; GERBRANDT, L. K., and PRIBRAM, K.: While monkey awaits: electrocortical events recorded during the foreperiod of a reaction time study. Electroenceph. clin. Neurophysiol. 31: 115–127 (1971).

GAZZANIGA, M. S. and HILLYARD, S. A.: Attention mechanisms following brain bisection; in KORNBLUM Attention and performance, vol. 4, pp. 221–238 (Academic Press, New York 1972).

GERBRANDT, L. K.; GOFF, W. R., and SMITH, D. B.: Distribution of the human average movement potential. Electroenceph. clin. Neurophysiol. 34: 461–474 (1973).

GILDEN, L.; VAUGHAN, H. G., and COSTA, L. D.: Summated human EEG potentials with voluntary movements. Electroenceph. clin. Neurophysiol. 20: 433–438 (1966).

GOFF, W. R.; MATSUMIYA, Y.; ALLISON, T., and GOFF, G. D.: Cross-modality comparisons of averaged evoked potentials; in DONCHIN and LINDSLEY Average evoked potentials. NASA SP-191, pp. 95–141 (US Government Printing Office, Washington 1969).

HÉCAEN, H. and AJURIAGUERRA, J. A. DE: Left-handedness: manual superiority and cerebral dominance (Grune & Stratton, New York 1964).

HILLYARD, S. A.: The CNV and human behavior: a review. Electroenceph. clin. Neurophysiol. Suppl. *33:* 161–171 (1973).

HILLYARD, S. A. and GALAMBOS, R.: Eye-movement artifact in the CNV. Electroenceph. clin. Neurophysiol. *28:* 173–182 (1970).

JARVILEHTO, T. and FRUHSTORFER, H.: Differentiation between slow cortical potentials associated with motor and mental acts in man. Expl Brain Res. *11:* 309–317 (1970).

KÖHLER, W. and O'CONNELL, D. N.: Currents of the visual cortex in the cat. J. cell. comp. Physiol. *49:* suppl. 2, pp. 21–43 (1957).

KÖHLER, W. and WEGENER, J.: Currents of the human auditory cortex. J. cell. comp. Physiol. *45:* suppl. 1, pp. 25–54 (1955).

KORNHUBER, H. H. und DEECKE, L.: Hirnpotentialänderungen bei Willkürbewegungen und passiven Bewegungen des Menschen. Bereitschaftspotential und reafferente Potentiale. Pflügers Arch. ges. Physiol. *284:* 1–17 (1965).

LOW, M. D.: in DONCHIN and LINDSLEY Average evoked potentials. NASA SP-191, pp. 163–171 (US Government Printing Office, Washington 1969).

LOW, M. D.; BORDA, R. P.; FROST, J. D., and KELLAWAY, P.: Surface negative slow potential shift associated with conditioning in man. Neurology, Minneap. *16:* 771–782 (1966).

LOW, M. D. and MCSHERRY, J. W.: Further observations of psychological factors involved in CNV genesis. Electroenceph. clin. Neurophysiol. *25:* 203–207 (1968).

MCADAM, D. W. and SEALES, D. M.: Bereitschaftspotential enhancement with increased level of motivation. Electroenceph. clin. Neurophysiol. *27:* 73–75 (1969).

MCADAM, D. W. and WHITAKER, H. A.: Language production: electroencephalographic localization in the normal human brain. Science *172:* 499–502 (1971).

MCCALLUM, W. C. and KNOTT, J. R. (eds): Event-related slow potentials of the brain. Electroenceph. clin. Neurophysiol. Suppl. *33:* 1–390 (1973).

MCCALLUM, W. C. and WALTER, W. G.: The differential effects of distraction on the contingent negative variation in normal and neurotic subjects. Electroenceph. clin. Neurophysiol. *25:* 319–329 (1968).

O'LEARY, J. L. and GOLDRING, S.: D-C potentials of the brain. Physiol. Behav. *44:* 91–125 (1964).

OTTO, D. A. and LEIFER, L. J.: The effect of modifying response and performance feedback parameters on the CNV in humans. Electroenceph. clin. Neurophysiol. Suppl. *33:* 29–37 (1973).

PICTON, T. W. and LOW, M. D.: The CNV and semantic content of stimuli in the experimental paradigm: effect of feedback. Electroenceph. clin. Neurophysiol. *31:* 451–456 (1971).

REBERT, C. S. and KNOTT, J. R.: The vertex non-specific evoked potential and latency of contigent negative variation. Electroenceph. clin. Neurophysiol. *28:* 561–565 (1970).

ROSEN, S. C.: Intersensory electrocortical conditioning of steady potential shifts in normal and epileptic monkeys; doctoral diss., New York (University Microfilms, Ann Arbor 1969).

SEMMES, J.: Hemispheric specialization: a possible clue to mechanism. Neuropsychologia 6: 11–26 (1968).

SPERRY, R. W.: Neurology and the mind-brain problem. Am. Sci. 40: 291–312 (1952).

STAMM, J. S. and ROSEN, S. C.: Electrical stimulation and steady potential shifts in prefrontal cortex during delayed response performance by monkeys. Acta Biol. exp., Vars. 29: 385–399 (1969).

STRAUMANIS, J. J.; SHAGASS, C., and OVERTON, D. A.: Problems associated with application of the contingent negative variation to psychiatric research. J. nerv. ment. Dis. 148: 170–179 (1969).

SUTTON, S.: The specification of psychological variables in an average evoked potential experiment; in DONCHIN and LINDSLEY Average evoked potentials. NASA SP-191, pp. 237–298 (US Government Printing Office, Washington 1969).

SYNDULKO, K.: Relationships between motor potentials and CNV. Electroenceph. clin. Neurophysiol. 27: 706 (1969).

SYNDULKO, K.: Cortical slow potential shifts in humans during sensory and motor tasks; doctoral diss., Los Angeles (University Microfilms, Ann Arbor 1972).

TECCE, J. J.: Contingent negative variation (CNV) and psychological processes in man. Psychol. Bull. 77: 73–108 (1972).

TECCE, J. J. and SCHEFF, N. M.: Attention reduction and suppressed direct-current potentials in the human brain. Science 164: 331–333 (1969).

VAUGHAN, H. G., jr.: The relationship of brain activity to scalp recordings of event-related potentials; in DONCHIN and LINDSLEY Average evoked potentials. NASA SP-191, pp. 45–94 (US Government Printing Office, Washigton 1969).
   Prog. clin. Neurophysiol., vol.1, Ed. J. E. DESMEDT, pp. 132–150 (Karger, Basel 1977)

WALTER, W. G.: Slow potential changes in the human brain associated with expectancy, decision and intention. Electroenceph. clin. Neurophysiol. Suppl. 26: 123–130 (1967).

WALTER, W. G.; COOPER, R.; ALDRIDGE, V. J.; McCALLUM, W. C., and WINTER, A. L.: Contingent negative variation: an electric sign of sensorimotor association and expectancy in the human brain. Nature, Lond. 203: 380–384 (1964).

WASMAN, M.; MOREHEAD, S. D.; LEE, H. Y., and ROWLAND, V.: Interaction of electrooocular potentials with the contingent negative variation. Psychophysiology 7: 103–111 (1970).

Dr. KARL SYNDULKO, Gateways Hospital, 1891 Effie Street, Los Angeles, CA 90026 (USA). Tel. (213) 666 0171.

# Event-Related Cerebral Potentials and the Initiation of Voluntary Contraction

Attention, Voluntary Contraction and Event-Related Cerebral Potentials.
Prog. clin. Neurophysiol., vol. 1, Ed. J. E. Desmedt, pp. 132–150 (Karger, Basel 1977)

## Cerebral Potentials and the Initiation of Voluntary Movement

Lüder Deecke and Hans H. Kornhuber

Department of Neurology, University of Ulm, Ulm

There are many experimental data about motor responses to electrical stimulation of different parts of the nervous system, the effects of lesions, and bioelectric potentials evoked by sensory stimuli, etc., but little is known about the processes underlying voluntary movement. Usually reference is made to the motor cortex if voluntary movements are discussed in contrast to reflex movements. However, it is clear that the motor cortex cannot by itself organize meaningful movements, since movements must be related both to internal stimuli signalling the needs of the organism as well as to external stimuli from the environment, and the motor cortex is not equipped with all the afferents necessary for this task. Other structures must be involved because many types of voluntary movement are possible in cats and monkeys after bilateral extirpation of the motor cortex [Bard, 1938; Hines, 1944].

For these reasons, it was decided in 1964 to investigate the cerebral potentials preceding voluntary (as opposed to reflex or conditioned) movements in man [Kornhuber and Deecke, 1964, 1965]. Earlier investigations of Bates [1951] had failed to detect cerebral potentials in man before the onset of voluntary movement, and Caspers' DC recording method without averaging did not show reliable potential changes preceding movement when recorded from the human scalp [cf. Caspers et al., 1963].

Therefore, a method of time reversed (opisthochronic) averaging of bioelectrical potentials was developed. With this method, three potentials with different distributions over the scalp and different time courses preceding voluntary finger movement could be distinguished [Deecke et al., 1969, 1973], while somewhat different potentials appeared before voluntary eye movements [BECKER *et al.,* 1968, 1972]. From these and other data, a more plausible theory of the neural organisation of voluntary movement has evolved [KORNHUBER, 1971, 1974a, b].

## Methods

Electrical potentials recorded from different positions on the human scalp (mono- and bipolar leads with a long time constant or DC recordings) were stored on magnetic tape together with a needle EMG of the moved limb, a strain gauge recorded mechanogram, the electrooculogram and the galvanic skin reflex for controls. By means of control experiments, care was taken to obtain the real start of movement in the effector muscles. Lid blinks and vertical eye movements were monitored by special leads. The first action potential of the electromyogram was used to start a quartz crystal clock which generated a second pulse after exactly 500 or 1,000 msec, respectively. This second pulse served as the trigger pulse to initiate the time-reversed averaging. By this procedure, the potentials preceding and following the onset of movement were obtained as a continuous graph. Trials containing artefacts due to head movements, lid blinks, galvanic skin reflex, etc. were eliminated by means of a careful editing procedure prior to averaging. Non-polarizable Ag/AgCl electrodes (Beckman) were used for recording. Linked ears, chin electrodes or extracranial electrodes (e.g. linked sternum-vertebra prominens), were used for reference.

## Potentials Preceding Voluntary Rapid Finger Movements

There are three potentials preceding voluntary rapid finger movements: Bereitschaftspotential (BP) or readiness potential (RP), pre-motion positivity (PMP) and motor potential (MP).

### Bereitschaftspotential

Contrary to our expectations and to classical theories on the role of the motor cortex in initiating movement, the first potential preceding voluntary finger movement is not unilateral (contralateral); instead, it is a *bilateral,* slowly increasing surface-negative potential which appears at the anterior parietal and precentral electrodes. On average, it starts about 0.8 sec prior to the onset of a rapid finger movement. The latency differs considerably between subjects, but is rather constant within subjects (fig. 1). The BP is maximal at the vertex, and it may be positive at frontal and basal leads. In the ipsilateral hemisphere, where the BP is not contaminated with the MP, it is slightly larger over anterior parietal than

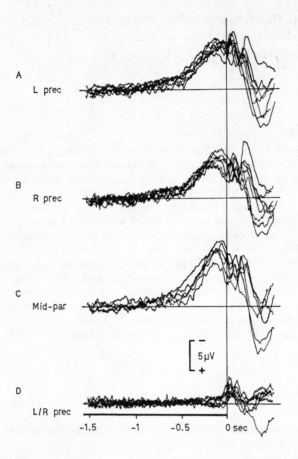

A
L prec

B
R prec

C
Mid-par

−
5 µV
+

D
L/R prec

−1.5      −1      −0.5      0 sec

*Fig. 1.* Cerebral potentials preceding voluntary finger movement. Superposition of the traces from 8 different experiments performed on different days of the same subject. Each trace represents the average of about 1,000 trials involving a rapid voluntary volar flexion of the *right* index finger. Negativity of the active electrode records upwards. The upper three groups of records represent recordings from left precentral (A), right precentral (B) or mid parietal (C) against linked ears reference. *D* Bipolar recording between the left (negative upwards) and the right precentral leads. The time is indicated in seconds along the abscissa, zero time representing the onset of the earliest EMG activity in flexor indicis muscle. The records disclose a high consistency and allow the identification of three components: (1) The negative BP or RP starting about 0.8 sec (onset time prior to first EMG activity) bilaterally over parietal and precentral regions. (2) The PMP, onset time 90–80 msec, also bilateral over parietal and precentral regions. (3) The negative MP, onset time 60–50 msec, unilateral, restricted to contralateral motor cortex, best seen in bipolar left versus right precentral recording.

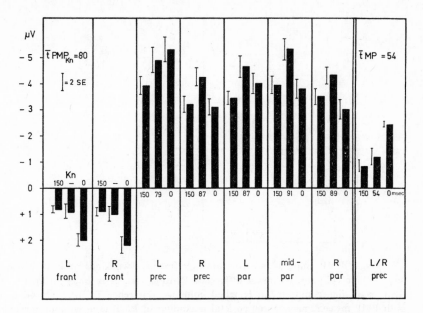

*Fig. 2.* Average amplitude of movement-related potentials at different electrode locations. From 87 experiments with right finger movements. Left columns of each group, potential 150 msec prior to first EMG activity, $BP_{150}$; center colums, potential at the kinking (reversal from negativity to positivity; fig. 1), $BP_{kn}$; right columns, potential at onset of EMG activity, $P_0$. Left of double line, monopolar recordings with frontal positive, at other locations negative potentials; the center columns represent the potential at the onset of the PMP; the onset times vary at different recording locations (mean PMP onset time 87 msec). Right of double line, bipolar recording left versus right precentral; the central column represents the potential at the onset of MP; mean onset time 54 msec. MP amplitude is the difference between center column and right column. From DEECKE *et al.* [1976].

over precentral electrodes, although the skull is slightly thicker over the parietal than over the precentral area, making the real difference even larger (fig. 2, 3). Measurements taken from 51 normal adult europide skulls (anatomical collection, University of Tübingen) revealed that skull thickness over the cortical hand area (1 cm anterior to $C_3$, $C_4$) averaged 4.67 mm, whereas at parietal electrode sites it averaged 5.24 mm. Thus, the bone is 11% thicker at parietal than at precentral electrode positions. On the other hand, in the mid-parietal ($P_z$) position bone is thinnest (5% thinner than precentrally) [DEECKE, 1973]. The amplitude of brain potentials, at least of the alpha rhythm, depends on skull thickness [LEISSNER *et al.*, 1970].

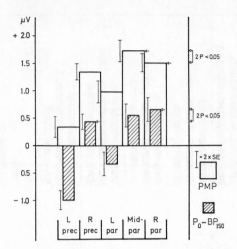

*Fig. 3.* PMP amplitudes across all experiments. Two kinds of PMP measurement: White columns, means of difference $P_0$-$BP_{kn}$ (fig. 2) in 87 experiments with right index finger movement. Hatched columns, difference $P_0$-$BP_{150}$. Positive up. Both PMP measurements show parietal maximum of PMP even without correction for different skull thickness (parietal thicker, see Methods). From DEECKE *et al.* [1976].

In experiments with several hundred finger movements, the amplitude of the average BP is $-5.3 \, \mu V$ (SD 2.3, SE 0.4), when recorded with a time constant of 1.2 sec. Considering a theoretical attenuation of 1/3 [cf. BECKER *et al.*, 1972], the DC amplitude would be $7 \, \mu V$. In the beginning of an experiment, the amplitude of the BP is usually larger. At parietal leads, the amplitude of the BP is exactly symmetrical over both hemispheres (bipolar recordings: left versus right parietal averaged 0), while over the precentral hand area it may begin to show a slight (although insignificant) asymmetry about 400 msec prior to onset of movement; this asymmetry (with the larger potential at the contralateral motor cortex) increases to a significant difference ($0.9 \, \mu V$) 150 msec prior to onset of movement in the EMG.

The BP belongs to the group of slow negative brain potentials (shifts of the cortical DC potential) and corresponds to a similar preparatory process as the contingent negative variation (CNV) recorded in conditioning experiments. However, there are four differences between the BP and the CNV: (1) The BP preceding simple fast finger movements has a parietal maximum while the CNV is maximal over frontal areas (see fig. 4 and

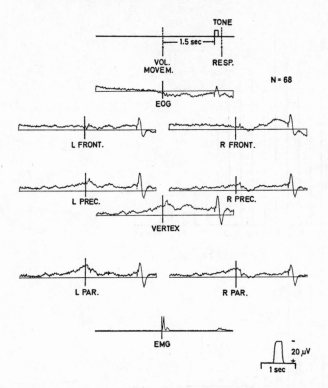

*Fig. 4.* Comparison of BP and CNV distribution in the same experiment. The subject performed voluntary (spontaneous, self-paced) standard right index finger movements at irregular intervals; this initated a delayed stimulus response program with a tone after a constant interval of 1.5 sec as the imperative stimulus, to which he responded with a second movement as fast as possible. BP maximal in parietal and vertex, absent in frontal leads; CNV maximal in frontal, absent in parietal leads. From an experimental demonstration at the 3rd CNV Conference, Bristol 1973. From DEECKE *et al.* [1976].

cf. JÄRVILEHTO and FRUHSTORFER, 1970). (2) The CNV is exactly bilaterally symmetrical – except if verbal stimuli or responses are involved [Low and Fox, 1977]; for the BP this is true only at parietal leads, while precentral leads usually have a slightly larger potential over the contralateral hemisphere in the last 300 or 400 msec prior to movement. (3) The BP increases gradually while the CNV increases more suddenly. (4) The BP is usually somewhat smaller than the CNV.

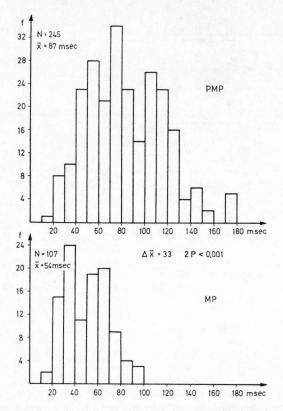

*Fig. 5.* Onset time distribution of PMP and MP with finger movement. Abscissae, onset time in msec prior to movement (first EMG activity in agonist muscle); ordinate, absolute frequency of occurrence. Onset time distributions of PMP from all precentro-parietal leads and of MP from bipolar left versus right precentral derivation are significantly different (2p<0.001, Wilcoxon test for paired differences). From DEECKE *et al.* [1976].

## Pre-Motion Positivity

The PMP is bilateral and widespread, like the BP; its onset time is 90–80 msec prior to the start of rapid finger movements as determined by the EMG (87 msec average, SD 34, SE 2.95). The PMP is a positive potential with the maximum at the mid-parietal electrode, where it averages +1.7 $\mu$V (SD 1.6, SE 0.28). A PMP appears in the majority (about two out of three) but not in all experimental subjects. Over the ipsilateral hemisphere (where it is not contaminated with the motor potential) the

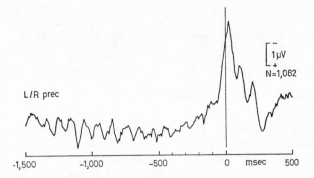

*Fig. 6.* Typical MP in bipolar left versus right precentral derivation. 1,082 movements of right index finger. O = Onset of movement (first EMG activity in right flexor indicis muscle). Note gradual upright deflection due to BP asymmetry (more negative left precentrally) beginning 400 msec prior to movement. MP onset about 60 msec. From DEECK *et al.* [1976].

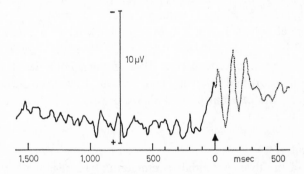

*Fig. 7.* Typical MP in bipolar derivation left precentral versus vertex. 295 movements of right index finger. O = Onset of a strain gauge recorded mechanogram. Note gradual downward deflection due to larger BP at the vertex. MP onset about 100 msec prior to mechanogram (corresponding to 67 msec prior to first action potentials in the agonist EMG). From KORNHUBER and DEECKE [1965].

PMP is significantly larger parietally than precentrally (fig. 3), although the skull is thicker over the parietal than over the precentral area.

Careful investigation of the first onset of muscle action potentials in the moving limb by means of bipolar needle electrodes (insulated except for the tip) has verified that the cortical PMP and the MP (see below) both occur *before* the onset of movement (see onset time histogram, fig. 5). There is some confusion in the literature regarding this point due

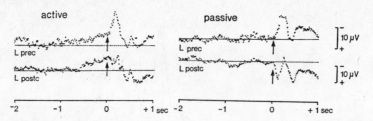

*Fig. 8.* Comparison of active with passive movements. Left: Potentials accompanying active voluntary rapid movements (combined flexion of the wrist and index finger), BP and (after movement onset) reafferent potentials. Right: Similar passive hand movements, showing only afferent potentials after the movement, but no BP. Monopolar recording from subgaleal Ag/AgCl needle electrodes versus nose. Note phase reversal around the rolandic fissure. From fig. 7C in KORNHUBER and DEECKE [1965].

to the fact that reafferent potentials (evoked by stimulation of receptors in the moving limb) were mistaken as the MP [cf. McADAM, 1973]. This explains the 'post-rolandic origin' and 'onset after movement' of GER-BRANDT's $N_2$ potential, which is not our MP [GERBRANDT *et al.*, 1971]. Probably the PMP is not just the decay of the BP, because there is no correlation between the amplitude of the BP and the amplitude of the PMP. Because of the short and relatively constant onset time, we suspect that the PMP reflects the cerebral process that corresponds to the actual command for the movement.

### *Motor Potential*

Only the last of the three potentials is unilateral. The negative MP is restricted to the contralateral precentral area. In the case of finger movement, its maximum is at the hand area of the motor cortex. It starts 60–50 msec prior to the onset of movement in the EMG (average 54 msec, SD 19, SE 3.1). It is best seen in bipolar leads of the contralateral versus ipsilateral precentral hand area (fig. 1, 6) or in bipolar leads of the contralateral precentral hand area versus the vertex (fig. 7), or versus frontal areas. Over the contralateral precentral hand area its average amplitude is 1.6 $\mu$V (SD 1.3, SE 0.1). The MP obviously corresponds to the discharge of neurons in the motor cortex preceding the type of movement that is strongly represented in motor cortex such as finger movement.

After the onset of movement in the EMG, a complex cortical potential appears which is also seen after passive movement of the same finger and hand (fig. 8) [KORNHUBER and DEECKE, 1965].

### Hemispheric Asymmetries of the Cerebral Potentials Preceding Voluntary Finger Movements Related to Handedness

Comparison of the cerebral potentials preceding right and left finger movements revealed, in first approximation, a mirror image-like behavior of the amplitudes of the BP (measured 150 msec prior to onset of movement) and of the MP (recorded with bipolar leads right versus left precentral motor hand area). However, on closer consideration, a group of 19 right-handed and 13 left-handed individuals showed that both the BP and the MP are significantly larger over the dominant hemisphere in right-handed individuals (irrespective of whether the movements of the contralateral or ipsilateral hand are under consideration). However, such a significant hemispheric difference does not exist in the left-handed individuals, although there was an analogous trend in the same direction (i.e. for left-handed individuals, the right hemisphere tended to have slightly larger potentials). This result corresponds to the fact that hemispherical lateralization is more pronounced in right-handed than in left-handed individuals.

### Cerebral Potentials Preceding Voluntary Saccadic Eye Movements in Man

The cerebral potentials preceding saccadic eye movements are similar to the potentials preceding rapid finger movements for the BP and the PMP (fig. 9) [BECKER et al., 1972], with the only exception that the PMP seems to start somewhat earlier preceding eye than preceding finger movements (fig. 9). However, in contrast to finger movements, there is no MP preceding saccadic eye movements. The positive spike at the onset of the movement, which originates in the region of the eyes, is probably of eye muscle origin (fig. 11E) [BECKER et al., 1972]. This oculomyogenic potential has been erroneously interpreted as a cortical MP by KURTZBERG and VAUGHAN [1973].

### Bereitschaftspotential and Attention

The amplitude of the BP is enhanced by attention. In experiments with a simple point on the one side and a table with letters on the other side of the visual field and the instruction to fixate each time another letter following the sequence of a code word, the BP was significantly larger preceding saccadic eye movements towards the table than preceding eye movements towards the simple point (fig. 10) [BECKER et al., 1972].

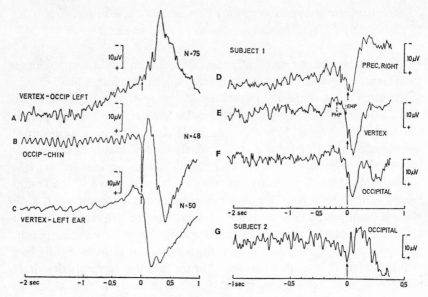

*Fig. 9.* Cerebral potentials accompanying voluntary eye movements (saccades). *A* BP preceding horizontal 40° eye movement to the left. Negative potential difference following the end of the movement due to larger positivity at the occipital lead. DC recording, N = 75. *B* Oculomyogenic potential at onset of eye movement to the right, positive evoked potential after the end of the movement. Time constant = 1.2 sec; N = 48. *C* BP and PMP preceding and EOG following eye movement to the right, time constant = 1.2 sec; N = 50. From BECKER *et al.* [1972]. *D, E, F* Subject 1, BP and typical PMP with onset at the upwards dotted arrow. The right precentral, vertex and occipital electrode locations are shown. Number of trials averaged = 45; time constant = 1.2 sec. The downward dotted arrow points to the small eye muscle potential (EMP). *G* Subject 2, PMP at mid-occipital electrode; not preceded by a BP. Number of trials averaged = 36. Same time constant. From BECKER *et al.* [1972].

The onset of the BP can be changed over a wide range by the experimental situation. If the experimental subject is asked to estimate a certain length of time starting from an auditory or visual signal and to execute the saccadic eye movement after this time, there is a close correlation between the duration of the waiting time and the duration of the BP (fig. 11A–D).

### Movement-Related Cerebral Potentials and Alpha Rhythm

There is no correlation of the average amplitude of BP, PMP, and MP with the average amplitude of the alpha rhythm. The movement-related

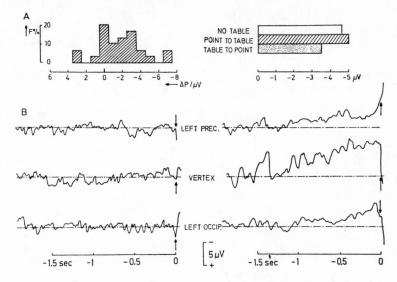

*Fig. 10.* BP and attention. *A* Left, percent frequency of occurrence of *ΔP* at the vertex. *ΔP* is the paired difference between BP preceding saccades towards a table with letters (see text) and BP preceding saccades to a simple point in the same experiment. Negative difference indicates larger BP preceding eye movement to the table. The difference is significant. Right, mean amplitudes of vertex BP in different experimental conditions. *B* Significantly larger BP with gaze towards the table with letters (right) than towards a simple point (left) in a typical experiment. N = 100; time constant = 1.2 sec. From BECKER *et al.* [1972].

potentials are of the same magnitude in subjects with a flat EEG as in subjects with a high amplitude alpha rhythm [DEECKE, 1973]. Furthermore, there is no relation of the phase of the alpha rhythm to the onset of voluntary finger movements (as was suspected by BATES), since the averaged alpha amplitude increases with

$$\overline{\sqrt{N}} \cdot \frac{\sqrt{\pi}}{2}$$

and not with $\sqrt{N}$ [KORNHUBER and DEECKE, 1965].

### Bereitschaftspotential Preceding Ramp and Step Movements

A recent theory of the neural organisation of voluntary movements [KORNHUBER, 1971, 1974a, b] postulates different function generators for fast (step, saccadic, or ballistic) movements which are thought to be preprogrammed, and for slow smooth continuous movements of voluntary

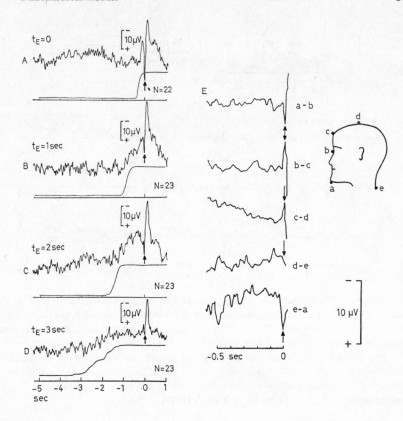

*Fig. 11. A–D* Effect of experimental situation on BP onset time. Subject was asked to wait a certain, self-determined time (time estimated = $t_E$) after target light onset in the peripheral field before starting the saccadic eye movement. Upper graphs in A to D, cerebral potentials in a vertex-chin-derivation; lower graphs, averaged current of target light bulb. The latter is increasingly smeared with increasing $t_E$ since the averaging process was triggered by the eye movement onset. BP duration correlates linearly with the length of the estimated times $t_E$. *E* Investigation of the oculomyogenic potential. Bipolar recordings in a sagittal line from chin (a), nasion (b) mid-frontal (c), vertex (d), and neck (e) revealed a potential reversal at the nasion and another more diffuse reversal between vertex and neck, suggesting intraorbital generation of the sharp oculomyogenic potential. Saccades to the left. N = 56. From BECKER *et al.* [1972].

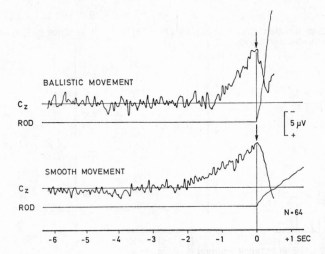

*Fig. 12.* Comparison of rapid and slow hand movements. The subject was pushing a rod into a tube at irregular intervals and varied the speed of the movement at random. BP preceding slow (smooth) movements (less than 10 cm/sec) starts significantly earlier and is usually larger than BP preceding rapid (ballistic) movement (more than 100 cm/sec). From BECKER *et al.* [1976].

speed (ramp movements). Therefore, the brain potentials preceding either slow or rapid hand movements have been studied comparatively [BECKER *et al.*, 1972]. The subjects were asked to hold the grip on the end of a rod, the elbow resting on a table for support and to push the rod into a tube at irregular intervals, varying the speed of these movements randomly. The rod and the tube served as a capacitative pickup for recording position and speed of movement. Movements below 10 cm/sec and above 100 cm/sec were electronically gated for analysis into the computer together with the corresponding brain potentials. The BP started about 0.8 sec prior to the onset of fast movement, whereas it preceded slow movements by 1.3 sec on the average (fig. 12). This onset time difference between slow and rapid movements is highly significant at all electrode positions (fig. 13). Furthermore, there was a significantly larger amplitude of the BP preceding slow than preceding rapid movements. The latency difference suggests that it might take more time to prepare for smooth than for a rapid movement. Therefore, the motor reaction times were measured for smooth and rapid movements upon an auditory stimulus

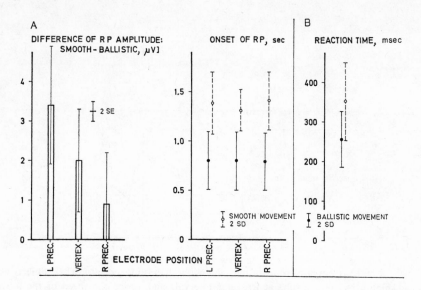

*Fig. 13.* Difference of BP preceding slow and rapid hand movement. *A* Left: The columns represent the difference of the BP amplitude preceding slow movements minus the BP amplitude preceding slow movement. Right: The onset times of BP preceding slow movement (open circles, top) are significantly longer than preceding rapid movement (filled circles). $C_3'$ and $C_4'$ are 1 cm anterior of the respective 10/20 positions, thus $C_3'$ is over the left, $C_4'$ over the right precentral hand area; $C_z$ at the vertex. *B* The reaction time to an auditory stimulus is significantly longer preceding slow than rapid movements. Ordinate: Time in msec between stimulus onset and movement onset. From BECKER *et al.* [1976].

given at irregular intervals, using the same setup as for the previously described experiments. Subjects were required to react as fast as possible to this command stimulus by pushing the rod into the tube, but varying the speed of movement randomly. In agreement with the longer BP, the motor reaction time to the auditory stimulus was significantly longer for slow ramp than for fast step movements (fig. 13B).

## Movement-Related Cerebral Potentials in Basal Ganglia Disease

In order to test the effect of basal ganglia disease on the three different potentials preceding voluntary finger movements, a study of 22 hemiparkinson patients was carried out [for details, see the paper of DEECKE *et al.*, this volume]. In agreement with the bilateral nature of the BP, this

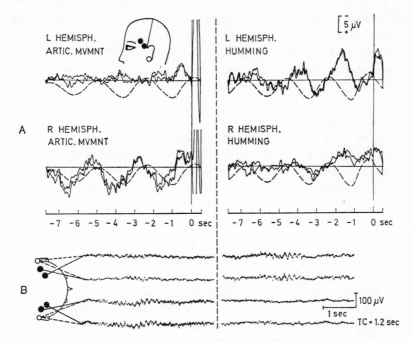

*Fig. 14.* Brain potentials related to respiration (R waves). *A* R waves preceding an articulatory movement of the mouth – forming a snout (left graphs) – are larger over the right hemisphere. R waves preceding humming of a tone (right graphs) are larger over the left hemisphere. *B* Original EEG recordings from the same experiment. The hemispherical asymmetries of the alpha and theta waves correspond to the R-wave asymmetries. The alpha and theta waves are smaller over the hemisphere with the smaller R waves. From GRÖZINGER *et al.* [1976].

potential was not only diminished unilaterally over the affected hemisphere, but was also diminished bilaterally preceding movements of the finger contralateral to the basal ganglia disease. The PMP, bilateral and widespread similar to the BP, is probably affected in a similar manner. Also the MP which is localized over the hand area of the precentral motor cortex was significantly smaller on the side of the affected basal ganglia than on the healthy side of the brain [cf. fig. 4a in DEEKE *et al.*, this volume].

### Cerebral Potentials Related to Respiration

Cerebral potentials related to respiration (R waves) have also been found, with frequencies around 0.25 Hz, which are contaminated with the

BP preceding the onset of vocalization or speech. These potentials (R waves) [cf. GRÖZINGER et al., 1974] do also accur in experiments without speaking, with a constant phase of respiration as the trigger. The R waves may show different amplitudes over both hemispheres. Usually, the more active hemisphere (which also shows smaller amplitudes of alpha or theta waves) has smaller R waves as well (fig. 14) [GRÖZINGER et al., 1974]. Galvanic skin reflex and other artefacts have been ruled out as the origin of the R waves. Epidural recording from cats demonstrated that the R waves are of intracranial origin. One possible origin of the R waves is cortical neuronal activity related to afferent or efferent respiratory discharge. Another possible origin are changes in cortical $CO_2$ concentration; it is known from animal experiments that changes in $pCO_2$ lead to changes of cortical DC potentials [CASPERS et al., 1963].

### Movement-Related Cerebral Potentials and Organization of Voluntary Movement

Since the movement-related potentials are (at least to a large extent) of cortical origin [McSHERRY et al., this volume], an attempt can be made to interpret these potentials with respect to theories of the organization of voluntary movement. The experimental data reported here are compatible with the theory which assumes that the motor commands of the cerebral cortex that result from information processing in sensory, association, and motivation areas must be converted by subcortical function generators into spatio-temporal motor patterns. These function generators are different for smooth continuous movements of voluntary speed (ramp movements) and for fast step movements. Presumably the fast (open-loop, saccadic, or ballistic) movements are preprogrammed by the cerebellum for timing and duration of activity, while the basal ganglia serve as the ramp generator. The cerebellum probably has two functions: (1) pulse generation and parametric gain adjustment for fast movements, and (2) hold regulation for positions between movements; the latter function is especially disturbed by lesions of the cerebellar nuclei.

For those movements that need sophisticated tactile analysis of objects (e.g. finger movements), the output patterns of the cerebellum and basal ganglia are further processed in the motor cortex [KORNHUBER, 1971, 1974a, b]. Between the onset of the PMP and the MP, there would be enough time for a loop from the sensory association areas via the cerebellum to the motor cortex following the well-known respective fiber tracts.

## References

BARD, P.: Studies on the cortical representation of somatic sensibility. Harvey Lect. *33:* 143–169 (1938).

BATES, J. A. V.: Electrical activity of the cortex accompanying movement. J. Physiol., Lond. *113:* 240–257 (1951).

BECKER, W.; DEECKE, L.; HOEHNE, O.; IWASE, K.; KORNHUBER, H. H. und SCHEID, P.: Bereitschaftspotential, Motorpotential und prämotorische Positivierung der menschlichen Hirnrinde vor Willkürbewegungen. Naturwissenschaften *55:* 550 (1968).

BECKER, W.; HOEHNE, O.; IWASE, K. und KORNHUBER, H. H.: Bereitschaftspotential, prämotorische Positivierung und andere Hirnpotentiale bei sakkadischen Augenbewegungen. Vison Res. *12:* 421–436 (1972).

BECKER, W.; IWASE, K.; JÜRGENS, R., and KORNHUBER, H. H.: Brain potentials preceding slow and rapid hand movements; in McCALLUM and KNOTT The responsive brain, pp. 99–102 (Wright, Bristol 1976).

CASPERS, H.; SCHÜTZ, E. und SPECKMANN, E. J.: Gleichspannungsveränderungen an der Hirnrinde bei Sauerstoffmangel. Z. Biol. *114:* 112 (1963).

DEECKE, L.: Die corticalen Potentiale des Menschen vor raschen willkürlichen Fingerbewegungen; Habilitationsschrift, Ulm (1973).

DEECKE, L.; BECKER, W.; GRÖZINGER, B.; SCHEID, P., and KORNHUBER, H. Human brain potentials preceding voluntary limb movements. Electroenceph. clin. Neurophysiol., suppl. *33:* 87–94 (1973).

DEECKE, L.; GRÖZINGER, B., and KORNHUBER, H. H.: Voluntary movement in man. Cerebral potentials and theory. Biol. Cybernet. *23:* 99–119 (1976).

DEECKE, L.; SCHEID, P., and KORNHUBER, H. H.: Distribution of readiness potential pre-motion positivity and motor potential of the human cerebral cortex preceding voluntary finger movements. Expl Brain Res. *7:* 158–168 (1969).

GERBRANDT, L. K.; GOFF, W. R., and SMITH, D. B.: Distributions of the human average movement potential. Electroenceph. clin. Neurophysiol. *34:* 461–474 (1973).

GRÖZINGER, B.; KORNHUBER, H. H.; KRIEBEL, J., and MURATA, K.: Cerebral potentials during respiration and preceding vocalisation. Electroenceph. clin. Neurophysiol. *36:* 435 (1974).

HINES, M.: Significance of the precentral motor cortex; in BUCY The precentral motor cortex, pp. 459–494 (University of Illinois Press, Urbana 1944).

JÄRVILEHTO, T. and FRUHSTORFER, H.: Differentiation between slow cortical potentials associated with motor and mental acts in man. Expl Brain Res. *11:* 309–317 (1970).

KORNHUBER, H. H.: Motor functions of the cerebellum and basal ganglia: the cerebello-cortical saccadic (ballistic) clock, the cerebello-nuclear hold regulator, and the basal ganglia ramp (voluntary speed smooth movement) generator. Kybernetik *8:* 157–162 (1971).

KORNHUBER, H. H.: Cerebral cortex, cerebellum and basal ganglia: an introduction to their motor function; in SCHMITT and WORDEN The neurosciences. Third Study Program, pp. 267–280 (MIT Press, Cambridge 1974a).

KORNHUBER, H. H.: The vestibular system and the general motor system; in KORN-
   HUBER Handbook of sensory physiology, vol. VI/2 (Springer, Berlin 1974b).

KORNHUBER, H. H. und DEECKE, L.: Hirnpotentialänderungen beim Menschen vor
   und nach Willkürbewegungen, dargestellt mit Magnetbandspeicherung und
   Rückwärtsanalyse. Pflügers Arch. ges. Physiol. 281: 52 (1964).

KORNHUBER, H. H. und DEECKE, L.: Hirnpotentialänderungen bei Willkürbewegungen
   und passiven Bewegungen des Menschen: Bereitschaftspotential und reafferente Potentiale. Pflügers Arch. ges. Physiol. 284: 1–17 (1965).

KURTZBERG, D. and VAUGHAN, H. G.: Electrocortical potentials associated with eye
   movements; in ZIKMUND The oculomotor system and brain functions. Smolenice
   Colloquium 1970, pp. 135–142 (Butterworths, London, and Slovak Academy
   of Sciences, Bratislava 1973).

LEISSNER, P.; LINDHOLM, L. E., and PETERSEN, I.: Alpha amplitude dependence on
   skull thickness as measured by ultrasound technique. Electroenceph. clin. Neurophysiol. 29: 392–399 (1970).

LOW, M. D. and FOX, M.: Scalp-recorded slow potentials asymmetries preceding
   speech in man; in DESMEDT Language and hemispheric specialization in man.
   Prog. clin. Neurophysiol., vol. 3 (Karger, Basel, in press 1977).

Prof. HANS H. KORNHUBER and Doz. Dr. L. DEECKE, Department of Neurology,
University of Ulm Medical School, 9 Steinhövelstrasse, D–79 Ulm (FRG). Tel.
(0731) 17 82 28.

Attention, Voluntary Contraction and Event-Related Cerebral Potentials.
Prog. clin. Neurophysiol., vol. 1, Ed. J. E. Desmedt, pp. 151–163 (Karger, Basel 1977)

# Cerebral Potentials Preceding Voluntary Movement in Patients with Bilateral or Unilateral Parkinson Akinesia

L. Deecke, H. G. Englitz, H. H. Kornhuber and G. Schmitt

Department of Neurology, University of Ulm, Ulm

The present study is not so much a clinical study aimed towards better understanding of the pathophysiology of Parkinson's disease, but rather attempts to gain further insight in the nature of the potentials preceding voluntary movement: Bereitschaftspotential (BP), pre-motion positivity (PMP) and motor potential (MP). These have been amply investigated in normal man [Kornhuber and Deecke, 1964, 1965; Vaughan et al., 1965; Gilden et al., 1966; Deecke et al., 1969, 1973, 1976] but lack so far lesion experiments which, in the human, can only consist of careful observation of diseases. Since the pre-movement brain potentials have been attributed to certain brain structures [Kornhuber, 1971, 1974; Deecke et al., 1973, 1976], it is necessary to study these potentials in patients with deficiencies of such structures.

As a first attempt, the commonest central motor disease, parkinsonism, was selected. This disorder appeared to be most appropriate for the study of pre-movement potentials, because it (1) is a well-defined lesion of an important central motor subsystem, the basal ganglia, and (2) has as its deficiency symptom (the release symptoms are tremor and rigidity) akinesia, an impairment of voluntary movement itself, with an almost complete abolition of all voluntary movement in the severe cases.

## Methods

Experiments were carried out in a total of 33 parkinsonian patients, in 22 of whom the disease was only unilateral. This condition will be called hemiparkinsonism here, although it mostly represented a unilaterally commencing parkinsonism, later also involving the other side. True (persisting) hemiparkinsonism is extremely rare.

The subjects reclined in an EEG chair and performed quick voluntary volar flections of the index finger by pulling the trigger of a pistol. An electric pulse was generated at the very first displacement of the pistol's trigger. The EMG of the right and left flexor indicis muscle was recorded, rectified and averaged, in order to determine the exact onset of movement in relation to the trigger pulse. Right and left index finger flections were investigated alternately in blocks of approximately 100 trials in the same experiment. The starting condition (first right, then left-sided movements and vice versa) was randomized in order to avoid trends. Totals of 400–500 movements of either side were averaged. During the experiment the subjects fixed their gaze on a given point. In addition, the vertically recorded electrooculogram was continuously monitored.

The experimenter could electrically mark all movements containing oculomotor and other artefacts which, on analyzing the tape-stored data in opposite time direction – reverse averaging [KORNHUBER and DEECKE, 1964] were excluded from the average.

The cerebral potentials were recorded monopolarly versus a linked ear reference, using Beckman electrodes attached with collodion to left, mid, and right precentral positions ($C_3'$, $C_z$, $C_4'$) and to left, mid, and right parietal positions ($P_3$, $P_z$, $P_4$). Positions $C_3'$ and $C_4'$ did not conform with the 10/20 system, but were placed to overlie the motor cortex hand area as described elsewhere [DEECKE et al., 1969]. In addition, bipolar recordings contralateral precentral versus ipsilateral precentral and versus vertex were used. Statistical analysis in the hemiparkinsonian patients was done using the $t$-test of paired differences, giving the opportunity to comparing the good with the affected side in the same individual and experiment. The bilateral parkinsonian patients were compared with a control group similar in age distribution and sex ratio (11 neurological patients without brain disorders, slipped discs, etc.).

## Results

### Bilateral Parkinsonism

In the bilateral parkinsonian patients considerably smaller and even positive BPs were observed. On average, the BP was abolished or rather slightly positive: The contralateral precentral BP, measured at the time of EMG onset ($P_0$), averaged +0.37 $\mu$V (SD 1.85, SE 0.58). In our normal subjects of previous experiments, the same amplitude averaged –5.3 $\mu$V (SD 2.9, SE 0.5) [DEECKE et al., 1973, 1976].

However, the average age of the parkinsonian patients of 65.6 years differed considerably from the one of our young normal students, and the BP has not been investigated so far in the aged. Therefore, the BP was studied in different age groups (the results will be reported elsewhere). The 11 oldest subjects (average age 60.2 years) constituted the control group for the 11 patients with bilateral parkinsonism. In these controls, the contralateral precentral BP at the time of movement onset, $P_0$, averaged $-2.64\,\mu V$ (SD 2.43, SE 0.73), which was significantly larger than in the parkinsonian group ($p<0.05$).

*Hemiparkinsonism*

For the 22 hemiparkinsonian patients no control group was necessary since each patient could serve as his own control by comparing the affected side with the healthy side. Hemiparkinsonian patients showed a significant reduction of the BP amplitude in leads contralateral to the akinetic side of the body on the same side as the basal ganglia disorder. This is in contrast to normal subjects, as seen in figure 1A, where the cerebral potentials preceding right-sided finger movement were compared with those preceding left-sided movement. In the normal subject, negativity was always larger at that precentral electrode, which was contralateral to the movement. Hence bipolar recordings left versus right precentral (bottom graphs of fig. 1A) were mirror images.

The situation was different in hemiparkinsonism, e.g. of the left side (fig. 1B). When the healthy (right) index finger was moved, the contralateral BP preponderance was markedly increased, yielding a pronounced deflection of the bipolar left versus right precentral derivation (bottom left). However, when the akinetic (left) finger was moved, the contralateral (affected) precentral region did not generate more negativity than the ipsilateral one. Both showed the same minimal BP, and in the bipolar recording the downward deflection to be expected from figure 1A bottom right did not occur.

This BP reduction over the affected hemisphere was statistically significant in the total of our 22 hemiparkinsonian patients (fig. 2A): the BP as measured 150 msec prior to the onset of movement ($P_{150}$) averaged $-2.3\,\mu V$ (SD 3.51, SE 0.74) over the healthy but only $-1.12\,\mu V$ (SD 2.76, SE 0.58) over the affected precentral region, when recorded contralaterally to the moving finger ($p<0.025$). The BP as measured at EMG onset ($P_0$) averaged $-4.21\,\mu V$ (SD 6.15, SE 1.31) over the healthy but only $-2.37\,\mu V$ (SD 3.95, SE 0.84) over the affected precentral region, when recorded contralaterally to the moving finger ($p<0.025$).

In figure 2A, the crossed (contralateral) situation was investigated: recording over the healthy hemisphere with movement of the healthy finger versus recording over the affected hemisphere with movement of the akinetic finger.

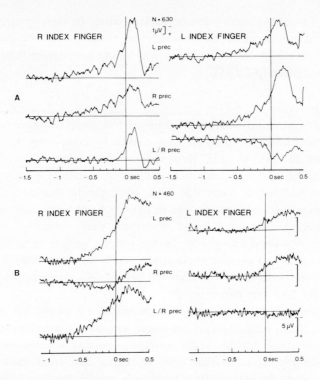

*Fig. 1.* Comparison of right and left-sided finger movements in a normal subject and in a hemiparkinsonian patient. *A* In the normal subject, negativity preceding movement is always larger in contralateral than in ipsilateral precentral leads
(contralateral preponderance of negativity). Thus, bipolar recordings left versus
right precentral (bottom graphs) are mirror images. Averages of 630 right-sided and
630 left-sided movements performed alternately in blocks of ca. 100 in the same experiment. *B* In a left-sided hemiparkinsonian patient, when moving the good (right)
finger, the contralateral preponderance of negativity is grossly enhanced, but it is
absent when moving the akinetic (left) finger. Thus, the downward deflection of *A*
bottom right is lacking, because the intact although ipsilateral precentral region generates as much negativity as the contralateral affected precentral region.

In figure 2B, the uncrossed (ipsilateral) situation was investigated:
healthy precentral region with movement of the akinetic finger ($P_{150}$ =
$-1.06 \mu V$, SD 3.35, SE 0.71; $P_0$ = $-2.45 \mu V$, SD 4.67, SE 0.99) versus
recording over the affected precentral region with movement of the
healthy finger ($P_{150}$ = $-1.28 \mu V$, SD 2.73, SE 0.58; $P_0$ = $-1.67 \mu V$, SD
3.12, SE 0.66). These differences were not significant ($p < 0.15$ and
$p < 0.45$).

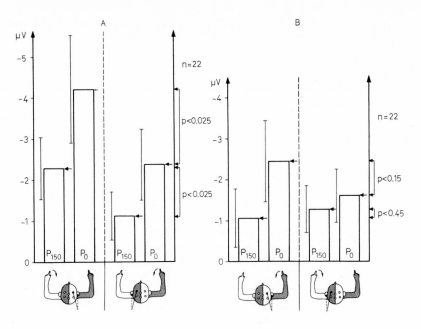

*Fig. 2.* Mean BP amplitudes of 22 hemiparkinsonian patients. *A* Contralateral situation: Recording over the good precentral region contralaterally to movement of the good finger (left side of *A*) versus recording over the affected precentral region contralaterally to movement of the akinetic finger. Two amplitude measurements: $P_{150}$ = BP amplitude measured (with respect to a prepotential baseline) at the time of 150 msec prior to movement onset in the EMG; $P_0$ = BP amplitude measured at the time of movement onset. In this and following figures schematic diagrams below the columns indicate: (1) recording location (here precentral versus linked ears; solid line, lead connected with A input; stippled line, lead connected with B input of differential EEG amplifier), and (2) side of movement (arrow at index finger). Hatching, affected hemisphere and contralateral akinetic arm; white area, good hemisphere and intact arm. On the left of each column, the double standard error (2 SE) is indicated. There is a significant reduction ($p<0.05$) of the two amplitudes over the affected hemisphere preceding movement of the akinetic finger (right side of *A*). *B* In the ipsilateral (uncrossed) situation, recording over the healthy precentral region with movement of the akinetic finger (left columns) versus recording over the affected hemisphere with movement of the good finger, no significant differences were found. This indicates that two effects are present (the effect of the hemisphere and the effect of the side of the body) which, in the ipsilateral situation, are superimposed, partially eliminating each other (fig. 3 shows the two effects in isolation).

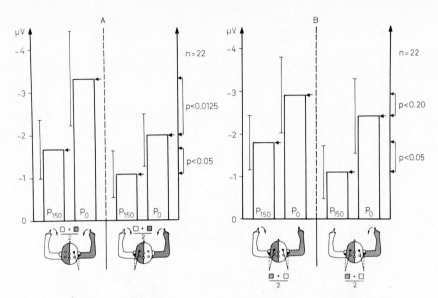

*Fig. 3.* BP in hemiparkinsonism: effect of the hemisphere and effect of the side of the body in isolation. *A* In order to get the effect of the hemisphere in isolation, the arithmetic mean was taken of the amplitudes recorded over the healthy precentral region with movements of the two sides: movement of the good finger + movement of the akinetic finger divided by 2 (left side of *A*). The same procedure with recording over the affected precentral region (right side of *A*) yielded significant reduction of the two amplitudes as indicated on the right. *B* In order to get the effect of the side of the body in isolation, the arithmetic mean was taken of the amplitudes recorded over the two precentral regions (affected precentral region + good precentral region divided by 2) with movement of the good finger (left side). This was compared with movement of the akinetic finger (right side), revealing a bilateral BP reduction (significant for the $P_{150}$ amplitude) preceding movement of the akinetic finger, which was also seen in midline leads (not shown).

If it were only the effect of the hemisphere causing BP reduction, such reduction should have been also present in the uncrossed (ipsilateral) situation. But it was not, at least not to a significant degree. It was, therefore, concluded that it is also the akinetic side of the body causing BP reduction and that in the uncrossed situation the two effects were superimposed and partially eliminated each other.

For the purpose of separating the two effects, the following calculations were done: In figure 3A, in order to get the effect of the hemisphere in isolation, the effect of the side of the body was eliminated by taking the arithmetic mean: movement of the healthy finger plus movement of the akinetic finger divided by 2. Significant differences were found (for $P_{150}$, $p<0.05$, for $P_0$, $p<0.0125$). The procedure to get the effect of the side of the body in isolation is described in figure 3B: Now, the arithmetic mean of the precentral recordings was taken (potential at the healthy precentral region plus potential at the affected precentral region divided by 2). Comparing with this procedure movement of the good finger with movement of the akinetic finger, we also found differences, significant at least for the $P_{150}$ amplitude, the BP proper ($p<0.05$).

In conclusion, besides the unilateral BP reduction over the affected hemisphere, we found a *bilateral* BP reduction when the akinetic finger was moved.

### The Two Other Potentials, PMP and MP

Whereas the MP could be readily evaluated in the bipolar recordings contralateral versus ipsilateral precentral or versus vertex, the PMP was difficult to record in the patients, because the typical potential course seen in the normal rarely occurred, which shows a definite kinking in the last 150 msec prior to movement in monopolar parietal and ipsilateral and sagittal precentral leads [cf. DEECKE et al., 1973, 1976]. Nevertheless, in the hemiparkinsonian patients an attempt was made to estimate also the PMP.

As PMP and MP are partially superimposed on each other, a 2-dimensional separation of the two potentials was tried: (1) *Spatial separation*. We measured the MP in leads, where it is most typical (bipolar recording: contralateral versus ipsilateral precentral or versus vertex) and the PMP where it is maximal, namely over the parietal region. (2) *Temporal separation*. PMP and MP have different onset times [fig. 5 in DEECKE and KORNHUBER, this volume], the PMP occurring on average 87 msec, the MP 54 msec prior to movement onset in the EMG. We therefore concluded that the PMP would be best described as $P_0-P_{90}$ in parietal leads, the MP as $P_0-P_{55}$ in bipolar leads contralateral versus ipsilateral precentral and versus vertex.

Highly significant differences were found for the MP (fig. 4A), proving that the MP is grossly reduced over the motor cortex on the side of the basal ganglia lesion. The evaluation of the PMP is more complicated because in the patients the potential difference $P_0-P_{90}$ or $P_0-P_{150}$ was not positive, as it was in the normal subjects [fig. 3 in DEECKE and KORNHUBER, this volume]. However, a rough estimation of the PMP seems possi-

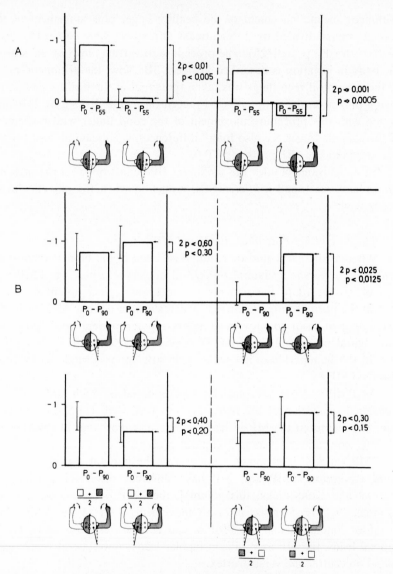

*Fig. 4.* MP and PMP in hemiparkinsonism (data of 22 patients; ordinates plotted in $\mu$V). *A* The MP in bipolar recording contralateral versus ipsilateral precentral (left side) and contralateral precentral versus vertex (right side) was grossly diminished, the latter was even positive, indicating more negativity at the vertex (input B of amplifier) than over the affected precentral region. $P_0$–$P_{55}$ is the difference between the amplitude measured at the time of movement onset in the EMG and the amplitude measured 55 msec prior to movement onset. The difference gives the

ble, if less negativity of the parietal $P_0-P_{90}$ difference is regarded as evidence for a larger PMP. Figure 4B upper left shows the contralateral situation, analogous to figure 2A. A trend can be seen towards more negativity (smaller PMP) on the affected parietal region preceding movement of the akinetic finger (right column). In the uncrossed situation of figure 4B upper right, analogous to figure 2B, there is a considerably smaller PMP (more negativity) with movement of the akinetic finger and with ipsilateral parietal recording, i.e. on the healthy side of the brain (right column).

This quite significant difference ($p < 0.0125$) suggests that for the PMP the effect of the side of the body is stronger than the effect of the hemisphere and, indeed, this was found after calculating the two effects in isolation, analogous to figure 3A and B.

In figure 4B lower right, showing the effect of the side of the body in isolation, a strong trend was found towards a smaller PMP (more negativity) with movements of the akinetic finger (right column). Calculating the effect of the hemisphere in isolation, as done in the lower left of figure 4B, no significant difference was found; even slightly more negativity (smaller PMP) occurred over the good parietal region. However, spread of negativity – contralateral preponderance (cf. fig. 1) and MP (cf. fig. 4A) – from the healthy precentral region towards the parietal lobe cannot be excluded. In summary, it seems clear that not only the BP is affected in parkinsonism, but also the two faster potentials PMP and MP.

In this context, it was of interest to know whether other brain potentials such as the alpha rhythm are also influenced by the disease. We

---

increase of negativity in the last 55 msec before movement. $P_{55}$ was chosen because the MP has an onset time of 60–50 msec in the normal subjects. *B* An attempt was made at estimating the PMP amplitude, although in the patients no positive parietal $P_0-P_{90}$ or $P_0-P_{150}$ differences could be found, contrary to normal [cf. fig. 3 in Deecke and Kornhuber, this volume]. Upper left: contralateral situation analogous to figure 2A, showing a trend towards more negativity (smaller PMP) over the affected parietal region preceding movement of the akinetic finger. Upper right: Ipsilateral situation analogous to figure 2B, showing a significantly smaller PMP (more negativity) preceding movement of the akinetic finger. This effect of the side of the body is seen at least as a trend in the lower right subfigure, where the effect of the side of the body in isolation is shown, analogous to figure 3B: bilateral reduction of PMP amplitude preceding movement of the akinetic finger. No marked effect of the hemisphere in isolation can be seen, analogous to figure 3A (lower left). Perhaps spread of negativity from the healthy precentral towards the healthy parietal region has influenced these results by adding additional negativity to the left column.

therefore compared the average alpha amplitude on the good hemisphere of our hemiparkinsonian patients with the one on the affected hemisphere. The two sides (good precentral region 98.4 $\mu$V, SD 37.5, SE 7.9 and affected precentral region 100.2 $\mu$V, SD 42.5, SE 9.1) were not significantly different but rather significantly equal ($2p<0.7$), proving that only the pre-movement potentials but not the EEG waves as such were depressed on the affected hemisphere of hemiparkinsonian patients.


## Discussion

Parkinson's disease is caused by a deficiency of the dopaminergic nigro-striatal system, whereby particularly the smooth ramp movements at voluntary speed are disturbed [KORNHUBER, 1971, 1974]. Akinesia is the difficulty to start a willed movement, although there is no paralysis. The present results show that the movement-related cortical potentials are affected in patients with parkinsonism. In bilateral parkinsonism, the BP was virtually abolished or rather slightly positive on average. In hemiparkinsonism, the BP was both *unilaterally* reduced in amplitude over the affected hemisphere (fig. 2A, 3A) and *bilaterally* reduced preceding movement of the akinetic finger (fig. 3B).

The two faster potentials PMP and MP, were also depressed. The MP was significantly smaller over the motor cortex on the affected side of the brain (fig. 4A). The PMP was difficult to evaluate because, contrary to our normal group of subjects, who showed positive $P_0$–$P_{150}$ differences [cf. fig. 3 in DEECKE and KORNHUBER, this volume], in most parkinsonian patients no definite kinking of the potential waveform occurred in the last 150 msec prior to movement onset.

The explanation for the absence of positive $P_0$–$P_{150}$ and $P_0$–$P_{90}$ differences in the patients (fig. 4B) is probably a different performance of the movement. Our trained young subjects were able to start an abrupt quick finger flexion out of complete muscular relaxation, which resulted in excellent triggering conditions. Furthermore, triggering on the EMG instead of using a mechanical device had already increased the frequency of occurrence of the PMP from 69% [DEECKE et al., 1969] to 85% of the subjects [DEECKE et al., 1976]. Undoubtedly, less accurate performance indeed to be expected in the patients, increases temporal jitter and is unfavorable for the recording of faster potentials such as PMP and MP.

Poorer performance has also to be expected for movement of the akinetic finger in the hemiparkinsonian patients. For a rough comparison, the latency between EMG onset and the trigger pulse on either side can be used. It was slightly longer with movement of the akinetic finger (30.8 msec, as opposed to 25 msec on the healthy side). The difference was not significant, but still an influence of performance on the PMP and MP side differences has to be discussed. For these reasons and due to the lack of positive $P_0$–$P_{90}$ differences, the present data are inappropriate for exact PMP measurements. Nevertheless, an attempt was made to enable arbitrary estimates, in that less negativity of the parietal $P_0$–$P_{90}$ amplitudes was regarded as evidence for a larger PMP and vice versa.

In the upper right of figure 4B, recordings over the ipsilateral parietal cortex with movement of the akinetic finger and of the healthy finger are compared. More negativity (smaller PMP) precedes movement of the akinetic finger (p<0.0125), and a trend for a bilateral PMP reduction preceding movement of the akinetic finger is seen in the lower right of figure 4B. This means that the PMP shows a similar behavior to the BP, at least with respect to the bilateral reduction preceding movement of the akinetic finger (effect of the side of the body). No marked effect of the hemisphere (upper and lower left of fig. 4B) can be seen. Spread of negativity from the healthy precentral region towards the ipsilateral parietal electrode could have added negativity to the left column in figure 4B lower left.

The most important result of the present investigation is the *bilateral* reduction of BP and PMP amplitudes preceding movement of the akinetic finger. As we have stressed since our early communications, preparation of a unilateral voluntary movement starts bilaterally and even bilateral-symmetrically. It remains bilaterally symmetric over the parietal region. Only in precentral leads, after ca. 400 msec before movement, a slight contralateral preponderance of negativity occurs and after 60 msec before movement the additional negativity of the MP can be seen. This bilateral occurrence of the BP and also of the PMP was in contrast to classical views, which were influenced by the common overestimation of the motor cortex with its unilaterally organized function [cf. DEECKE and KORNHUBER, this volume]. However, the motor cortex comes into play only later in the preparation of a voluntary movement, since the corresponding potential, the MP, starts about 60–50 msec prior to EMG onset. The MP is the only unilateral pre-movement potential. Movement design and priming command, however, are obviously not elaborated by the motor cortex but bilaterally by other cortical regions [KORNHUBER, 1971, 1974].

On the basis of the bilateral nature of BP and PMP, the bilateral reduction of the two potentials preceding movement of the akinetic finger
can be well understood. In unilateral cortical lesions, the readiness potential was found reduced unilaterally over the lesioned hemisphere [SHIBA-
SAKI, 1975]. Whether there was bilateral reduction with movement of the
paretic hand was not reported, but would be of interest.

In basal ganglia disorder, such as parkinsonism, particularly the slow
smooth movements are impaired, e.g. turning in bed, standing up, etc. In
the present investigation, the cortical pre-movement potentials were found
impaired preceding quick movements, for which the cerebellum rather
than the basal ganglia serves as the respective movement generator [cf.
KORNHUBER, 1971, 1974; DEECKE and KORNHUBER, this volume]. Possible explanations could be the impaired coordination between slow and
rapid movements, a diminished synaptic drive and/or transneuronal degeneration secondary to the basal ganglia disorder.

## Summary

Cerebral potentials preceding voluntary rapid finger movements were studied
in 33 cases of bilateral and unilateral parkinsonism, selected for marked akinesia
and minimal tremor. Right and left index finger movements were compared in the
same experiment. In the 11 bilateral patients, the Bereitschaftspotential (BP) or
readiness potential was bilaterally abolished or even slightly positive (mean contralateral precentral amplitude $+0.37$ $\mu$V, SD 1.85, SE 0.58), as opposed to 11 normal
individuals of a comparable age ($-2.64$ $\mu$V, SD 2.43, SE 0.73; $p < 0.05$).

In the 22 unilateral cases, a significant reduction ($p < 0.025$) of the BP amplitude was found on the affected side of the brain, i.e. contralateral to the akinetic
side of the body. The side of the larger BP did, therefore, not depend on the side of
the movement as in the normal, but on the side of the basal ganglia disorder. In addition to this unilateral diminution, there was a bilateral BP reduction preceding
movement of the akinetic finger.

The motor potential (MP) which in the normal is a unilateral negative potential with an onset time of 60–50 msec prior to movement onset over the contralateral motor cortex, was significantly smaller ($p < 0.0005$) preceding movement of the
akinetic finger recorded over the contralateral motor cortex on the side of the basal
ganglia disorder in bipolar contralateral versus ipsilateral precentral or versus vertex derivations.

The pre-motion positivity (PMP) appeared to be affected in a similar manner
as the BP, the bilateral reduction with movement of the akinetic finger being even
more pronounced.

*References*

DEECKE, L.; BECKER, W.; GRÖZINGER, B.; SCHEID, P., and KORNHUBER, H. H.: Human brain potentials preceding voluntary limb movements. Electroenceph. clin. Neurophysiol. Suppl. *33:* 87–94 (1973).

DEECKE, L.; GRÖZINGER, B., and KORNHUBER, H. H.: Voluntary finger movement in man. Cerebral potentials and theory. Biol. Cybernet. *23:* 99–119 (1976).

DEECKE, L.; SCHEID, P., and KORNHUBER, H. H.: Distribution of readiness potential, pre-motion positivity, and motor potential of the human cerebral cortex preceding voluntary finger movements. Expl Brain Res. *7:* 158–168 (1969).

GILDEN, L.; VAUGHAN, H. G., and COSTA, L. D.: Summated human EEG potentials with voluntary movements. Electroenceph. clin. Neurophysiol. *20:* 433–438 (1966).

KORNHUBER, H. H.: Motor functions of cerebellum and basal ganglia: the cerebellocortical saccadic (ballistic) clock, the cerebellonuclear hold regulator, and the basal ganglia ramp (voluntary speed smooth movement) generator. Kybernetic *8:* 157–162 (1971).

KORNHUBER, H. H.: Cerebral cortex, cerebellum, and basal ganglia: an introduction to their motor functions; in SCHMITT and WORDEN The neurosciences. Third Study Program, pp. 268–280 (MIT Press, Cambridge 1974).

KORNHUBER, H. H. und DEECKE, L.: Hirnpotentialänderungen beim Menschen vor und nach Willkürbewegungen, dargestellt mit Magnetbandspeicherung und Rückwärtsanalyse. Pflügers Arch. ges. Physiol. *281:* 52 (1964).

KORNHUBER, H. H. und DEECKE, L.: Hirnpotentialänderungen bei Willkürbewegungen und passiven Bewegungen des Menschen: Bereitschaftspotential und reafferente Potentiale. Pflügers Arch. ges. Physiol. *284:* 1–17 (1965).

SHIBASAKI, H.: Movement-associated cortical potentials in unilateral cerebral lesions. J. Neurol. *209:* 189–198 (1975).

VAUGHAN, H. G.; COSTA, L. D., and RITTER, W.: Topography of the human motor potential. Electroenceph. clin. Neurophysiol. *25:* 1–10 (1968).

Doz. Dr. LÜDER DEECKE and Prof. H. H. KORNHUBER, Department of Neurology, University of Ulm Medical School, 9 Steinhövelstrasse, *D–79 Ulm* (FRG). Tel. (0731) 17 82 28.

Attention, Voluntary Contraction and Event-Related Cerebral Potentials.
Prog. clin. Neurophysiol., vol. 1, Ed. J. E. DESMEDT, pp. 164–173 (Karger, Basel 1977)

# Voluntary Movement-Related Slow Potentials in Cortex and Thalamus in Man[1]

E. GROLL-KNAPP, J. A. GANGLBERGER and M. HAIDER

Institute of Hygiene and Department of Neurosurgery,
University of Vienna, Vienna

Following the description of the contingent negative variation (CNV) or expectancy wave (E wave), consisting of a slow negative potential shift in the brain, dependent on forming an association between paired stimuli of which the second is imperative, by WALTER et al. [1964], a similar phenomenon, associated with randomly performed voluntary movement was first described by KORNHUBER and DEECKE [1965] and has been termed motor Bereitschaftspotential (see this volume). In 1967, our team started to investigate the thalamo-cortical and cortico-thalamic interrelationships of these slow potential changes on non-sedated patients, undergoing stereotactic surgery whenever state and consent of the subject permitted it. In comparison to studies with chronically indwelling electrodes, the acquisition of data in acute stereotactic surgery required a greater number of subjects since the number of applied cortical and subcortical electrodes is limited. Earlier reports of our work were given by GANGLBERGER et al. [1968], GROLL-KNAPP et al. [1970] and HAIDER et al. [1968, 1969, 1972]. In our early work, the conclusion was drawn that thalamic structures are involved in the initiation of the slow potential phenomena on motor and pre-motor cortex. To our satisfaction, animal experiments of CHIORINI [1969], FUSTER and UYEDA [1971], SKINNER [1971] and REBERT [1972, 1973] are in favour of our early conclusions [cf. YINGLING and SKINNER, this volume].

[1] This work was supported by the Austrian fund for the advancement of scientific research.

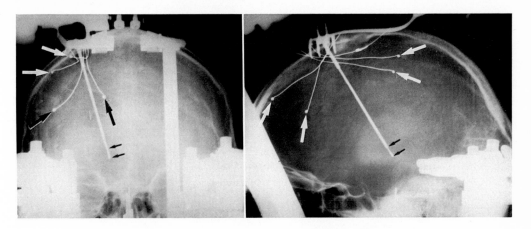

*Fig. 1.* Left: a-p; right: lateral X-ray exposure. The blunt arrows point to the subdural cortical electrodes, the other arrows indicate the two poles of the thalamic depth electrode. Tip is located in the V.c.pc (posterior basal portion of VP).

## Method and Material

The determination of the thalamic (or other) target point was performed according to the method of HASSLER [1959]. A stereotactic equipment, described by RIECHERT and MUNDINGER [1955] was used. The depth electrode, a coaxial probe with two poles separated by a distance of 5 mm, was inserted through high-frontal trephine hole. Through the same bore hole four flexible teflon-isolated silver-silverchlorid electrodes, with the tips fused into small globules, were introduced subdurally. The intention was to place two of them over the prefrontal cortex and two others over premotor and motor areas of the cortex. Since special care had to be taken so that no vascular damage be done, the exact placement of these cortical electrodes remained more or less a function of chance. The exact locations of depth and cortical electrodes were then confirmed on bi-dimensional X-ray exposures. In figure 1, an example of thalamic depth electrode, and cortical surface electrode position is shown. Additional vertex-mastoid electrodes were applied. For determination of polarity, the linked mastoid-reference was used. An overall distribution of recording sites from our last 50 cases is included in figure 5.

The majority of our cases were suffering from Parkinson's disease. Some are cases of extrapyramidal motor disturbances or cases of temporal lobe epilepsy. Also included are psychosurgical operations and thalamic interventions against intractable pain. Electrophysiological recordings and analyses of different phenomena were performed in 234 cases. In the last 50 of these, besides other phenomena, the slow potential changes related to voluntary movement were studied. The distribution of indications and target points of these patients is shown in table I. The nomenclature of HASSLER [1959] and the stereotactic atlas of SCHALTENBRAND and BAILEY [1954] are used.

*Table I.* Indications for stereotactic surgery and target points of the 50 cases included in this study

| Indications | Target point | Number of cases |
|---|---|---|
| Parkinson's disease | motor thalamus: V.o.a., V.o.p., zona incerta | 18 |
| Other extrapyramidal motor disturbances | V.o.a., V.o.p., L.po. | 4 |
| Intractable pain | V.c.pc., Ce. Tr. spinothal. | 12 |
| Temporal lobe epilepsy | Fx + CA, Am. m. orl. | 9 |
| Psychosurgery | M. fa. p., Am. m. | 7 |

The task requested from the subject was to press a button at irregular self-chosen intervals with the contralateral thumb in respect to the site of the target. The button switch was connected to a trigger device providing a marking signal on a 14-channel FM magnetic tape recorder and at the same time starting the average analogue computer in the mode of the so-called instantaneous opisthochronic analysis. The EEG was fed into a Correlatron 4096, the tape speed set so as to cause a delay of 2.335 sec, the total analysis time fixed on 4 sec.

## Results

Extracted from the mosaic pattern of the individual data the following common features can be described. The vertex-mastoid and vertex-bimastoid leads demonstrated the well-known pattern of the motor readiness potential (motorisches Bereitschaftspotential) as described by KORN-HUBER *et al.*

On the cortex, a variety of different patterns of slow potential changes was found. The differences seemed to be related to the varying electrode positions. In the following, we shall try to group some of the characteristic patterns according to their origin from certain cortical areas. Some motor readiness potentials similar to the ones from scalp derivations described in the literature have been found over the area 6a alpha and 6a beta of VOGT and VOGT [1926]. Examples from different sub-

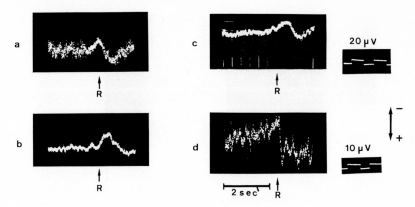

*Fig. 2.* Motor readiness potential from areas 6a alpha and 6a beta. *a* From an epileptic case. *b, c* Parkinson's disease. *d* Psychosurgery.

jects are shown in figure 2. All cases showed some slowly increasing negativity, the peak latency of which displayed great variations. One reason for this variation may be the kind of disturbance of the patient undergoing stereotactic surgery, another one the slight variation of electrode sites. The second and third (b+c) curve in figure 2 reached their peak latency long after the time of the trigger mark as caused by the pressing of the button with the contralateral thumb. These samples were from subjects suffering of Parkinson's disease. The start of the slowly rising negativity was rather late in these cases. A pre-motion positivity was sometimes seen just before the reaction. In all derivations from premotor cortex, a clearly defined positivity developed after the motor performance.

The few cases in which one electrode could be placed over the proper motor cortex (area 4) displayed a completely different picture. One sample is demonstrated in figure 3. There was almost no or only a hint of a slow negative shift, but a fast prominent positive decline started already before the actual movement, especially when the cortical electrode was placed on the cortical representation of arm or hand. In the prefrontal and fronto-polar areas (9, 10), the monopolar leads againts the linked mastoid very often showed little or no characteristic potentials at all. Surprisingly, relatively close-spaced bipolar leads sometimes revealed a very early and prominent slow potential shift, long before the motor action or

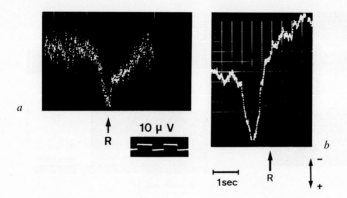

Fig. 3. *a* Motor potential from motor cortex (area 4). *b* Slow potential change at fronto-polar region (area 10).

already declining at the time of the action. One extreme example is given in figure 3.

While recordings from cortical electrodes showed relatively great differences between individuals with comparable electrode positions, this difference was of much lesser degree in the depth records.

In figure 4, typical traces of average motor readiness potentials from various thalamic nuclei and other subcortical structures are demonstrated. It is possible to record slow potentials associated with motor action from different specific and non-specific nuclei of the thalamus. As a common characteristic, they show a slowly rising negativity, starting before the motor action. There is not only a difference in amplitudes, but a marked one of peak latencies between the various nuclei. In the nc. medialis or dorsomedialis in all our cases a motor readiness potential was found, sometimes much more prominent (schematic presentation in fig. 5) as the sample in figure 4. A similar form of potential was encountered in the non-specific nc. centralis (centre médian of Luys).

In the specific motor relay nuclei (V.o.a., V.o.p.) and the subjacent zona incerta, the negativity seemed to start rather shortly before the motor action, but with a relatively sharp increase. It reached its peak invariably after the trigger mark produced by the thumb press. In this connection, it has to be considered that all recordings from specific motor relay nuclei were derived from subjects with Parkinson's disease or other extrapyramidal motor disturbances, who are slowed in their motor action due to their specific disease.

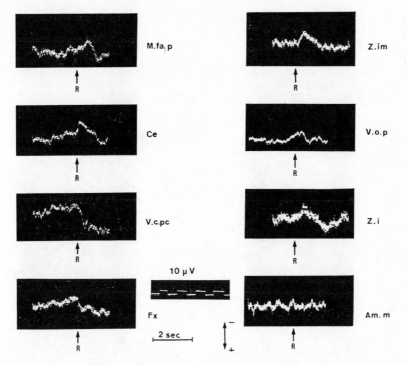

*Fig. 4.* Motor readiness and motor potentials from various thalamic nuclei and other subcortical structures. M.fa.p = Medialis fasciculosus posterior; Ce = nc. centralis or centre médian of Luys; V.c.pc = ventrocaudalis parvocellularis; Fx = fornix; Z.im = nc centralis intermedius; V.o.p = ventro-oralis posterior; Z.i = zona incerta; Am.m = nc. medialis Amygdalae. The different beginning of the traces is due to the different tape speeds during the intantaneous opisthochronic analysis.

The slow potential changes in the basal posterior portion of the specific sensory relay nucleus (V.c.pc., termination of the spinothalamic tract) showed as a most marked feature a sharp positive decline shortly after the motor action. In most cases, the slow motor potential changes recorded from the columna fornicis and neighbouring septal region showed a similarity to such ones recorded from the thalamus in the slowly rising part; but they are lacking the sharp increase of negativity shortly before and during the movement. They rather showed a similarity to the sharp positive decline after the motor action as in the sensory relay nuclei.

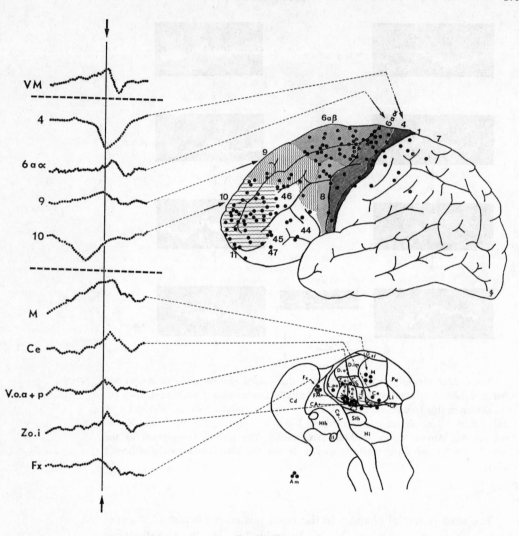

*Fig. 5.* Synoptic schematic presentation of movement-related slow potentials from different cortical and thalamic electrode positions.

On the contrary, the nc. amygdalae showed no slow potentials at all. As all stereotactic interventions on the amygdalum in our cases were secondary to fornico- and anterior commissurotomy, we cannot state whether this is a specific feature of the amygdalum or due to the previous operation.

In figure 5, a synoptic schematic presentation of recording sites of cortex, thalamic and other subcortical structures is shown together with typical slow potential changes related to voluntary movement. Here, the time relationship of different recording sites to the trigger mark of the motor performance can be clearly observed. The traces are drawn from original potentials composed from different patients. It must be stated in this connection that in a small percentage of patients no characteristic potentials were detectable. The stress of the situation of acute stereotactic surgery may be one of the reasons for this fact.

Figure 5 shows clearly that early slow potential changes long before the movement seem to occur mainly in the prefrontal and fronto-polar regions and also in the nc. medialis or dorsomedialis thalami. Shortly before the movement, additional sharp rises occur in the specific thalamic motor relay nuclei. Around the same time before and at the time of the movement in the proper cortical motor region a prominent sharp potential decline is found. After the motor action, the thalamic potentials reach their peak.

### Discussion

According to the results of our investigations, there seems to be at least four patterns of voluntary movement-related slow potential changes: One early marked positive shift in the fronto-polar and prefrontal cortical region and in the connected nc. medialis thalami. A slow negative potential change starting with some delay and a longer build-up until the time of the movement, occurring on the pre-motor region as well as in some thalamic nuclei. In the motor thalamus, an additional sharp rise in the negativity occurs shortly before the movement. Finally, in the proper motor region, a marked positive shift is encountered around the time of the movement. The time relationship of these four patterns of voluntary movement-related slow potential changes seems to indicate that decision and design of movement is started in the thalamo-prefrontal system and from there a motor readiness potential is initiated on premotor cortex and in different subcortical structures.

There seems to be an indication for a thalamo-cortical relationship for the process of coding and control of the outgoing message to the spinal cord. Electrophysiological correlates of this process seem to be the additional thalamic sharp rises of negativity together with the sharp positive decline on the proper motor cortex starting shortly before the movement, reaching its peak at the time of or shortly after the motor performance. In the specific sensory relay nuclei, a sharp decline of potential after the movement is encountered. These phenomena as well as similar potential changes in the fornix may be related to reafferent signals from the periphery.

Our results differentiate the common pattern emerging from the study with scalp electrodes in humans. These phenomena, as described by different authors, are probably an integration of the various cortical and subcortical mechanisms found in our study based on acute stereotactic surgery in humans.

## References

FUSTER, J. M. and UYEDA, A.: Reactivity of limbic neurons of the monkey to appetitive and adverse signals. Electroenceph. clin. Neurophysiol. *30:* 281–293 (1971).

CHIORINI, R.: Slow potential changes from cat cortex and classical aversive conditioning. Electroenceph. clin. Neurophysiol. *26:* 399–406 (1969).

GANGLBERGER, J. A.; GROLL-KNAPP, E. und HAIDER, M.: Stereotaktische Hirnoperationen und neuropsychologische Forschung. Dt. Ges. Psych. *26. Kongr., Göttingen 1968.*

GROLL-KNAPP, E.; GANGLBERGER, J. A., and HAIDER, M.: Relations between thalamic cortical and subperiosteal derivations of expectancy waves and orienting potentials. Electroenceph. clin. Neurophysiol. *28:* 322–325 (1970).

HAIDER, M.; GANGLBERGER, J. A., and GROLL-KNAPP, E.: Computeranalyzed thalamic potentials and their relation to expectancy waves in man. Acta neurol. latinoamer. *14:* 132–137 (1968).

HAIDER, M.; GANGLBERGER, J. A., and GROLL-KNAPP, E.: Thalamo-cortical components of reaction time. Acta psychol. *30:* 378–381 (1969).

HAIDER, M.; GANGLBERGER, J. A., and GROLL-KNAPP, E.: Computer analyis of subcortical and cortical evoked potentials of slow potential phenomena in humans. Confinia neurol. *34:* 224–229 (1972).

HASSLER, R.: Anatomie des Thalamus – Anatomy of the thalamus; in SCHALTENBRAND und BAILEY Einführung in die stereotaktischen Operationen mit einem Atlas des menschlichen Gehirns, vol. 1, pp. 230–290 (Thieme, Stuttgart 1959).

KORNHUBER, H. H. and DEECKE, L.: Hirnpotentialänderungen bei Willkürbewegungen und passiven Bewegungen des Menschen. Bereitschaftspotential und reafferente Potentiale. Pflügers Arch. ges. Physiol. *284:* 1–17 (1965).

REBERT, C. S.: Cortical and subcortical slow potentials in the monkey's brain during a preparatory interval. Electroenceph. clin. Neurophysiol. *33:* 389–409 (1972).

REBERT, C. S.: Elements of a general cerebral system related to CNV genesis in event-related slow potentials of the brain. Electroenceph. clin. Neurophysiol. Suppl. *33* (1973).

RIECHERT, T. und MUNDIGER, F.: Beschreibung und Anwendung eines Zielgerätes für stereotaktische Hirnoperationen (II Modell). Acta neuroclin., suppl. III, pp. 308–337 (1955).

SKINNER, J. E.: Abolition of a conditional surface-negative cortical potential during cryogenic blockade of the non-specific thalamo-cortical system. Electroenceph. clin. Neurophysiol. *31:* 197–209 (1971).

VOGT, C. und VOGT, O.: Die vergleischend-architektonische und die vergleischend-reizphysiologische Felderung der Grosshirnrinde unter besonderer Berücksichtigung der menschlichen Naturwissenschaften *14:* 1190–1194 (1926).

WALTER, C.; COOPER, R.; ALDRIDGE, J.; McCALLUM, C., and WINTER, L.: Contingent negative variation. An electric sign of sensomotor association and expectancy in the human brain. Nature, Lond. *203:* 380–384 (1964).

WALTER, G.: Slow potential changes in the human brain associated with expectancy, decision and intention in the evoked potentials. Electroenceph. clin. Neurophysiol., suppl. *26:* 123–130 (1967).

Dr. E. GROLL-KNAPP, Institut für Umwelthygiene, University of Vienna, 15, Kinderspitalgasse, *A–1095 Vienna* (Austria). Tel. (302) 43 15 45.

Attention, Voluntary Contraction and Event-Related Cerebral Potentials.
Prog. clin. Neurophysiol., vol. 1, Ed. J. E. DESMEDT, pp. 174–188 (Karger, Basel 1977)

# Analysis of Movement Potential Components

L. K. GERBRANDT

Department of Psychology, California State University, Northridge, Calif.

The cerebral potentials associated with abrupt, voluntary movements have been termed motor potentials by VAUGHAN et al. [1968] who suggested that all components of the movement-related potential (MP) are generated within the precentral gyrus, and are motoric potentials, having to do with the control and feedback to the pyramidal tract movement system. Other MP investigators [cf. DEECKE and KORNHUBER, this volume] recognize that both nonmotoric and motoric wavelets exist within the MP, but still interpret MPs as if they can be recorded as isolated components, each having a singular functional origin. In this chapter, the case is developed for dropping the specific term 'motor potential' in favor of the more general term *movement potentials*. Specifically, the point will be made that there are more than four MPs, some are asymmetrical and some are not, and that there are probably several nonmotoric MP components which are overlapping in their distributions with motoric MP components. It will be noted that failure to recognize these multiplicities of superposition of MP components has led [GERBRANDT et al., 1973] and will lead to unneeded controversies.

## Slow Potential Components

The first premovement potentials to be seen in the MP waveform are the slow potential components. These components, and the ways we have measured them [GERBRANDT et al., 1973], are labelled as 'N1' in figure 1. These recordings were made in 5 subjects over the presumed motor cortex contralateral to movement (0%); the position of the electrode locations are shown in comparison to 10–20 System. The N1 amplitudes at each of 12 electrode sites are averaged over the 5 subjects and plotted as a percentage of the site showing the largest N1 amplitude in figure 2. Notice that N1 is actually a positive rather than a negative slow potential over the presumed frontal cortex. This same finding is reported by VAUGHAN et al. [1968] and DEECKE et al. [1969]. Such a pattern might be produced by the summation of slow potentials generated in the frontal cortex with additional slow potentials generated more posteriorly in the Rolandic cortices. The lack of an asymmetry of the positive but not the negative slow components (fig. 2) indicates that these polarity reversals probably do not arise as a function of a single dipole oriented parallel to the skull surface.

Another indication of the multiple origins of slow potential MP components is the change in N1 asymmetry as a function of several variables. Notice in figures 2 and 3 that a larger asymmetry is present over the presumed motor cortex (0%), compared to presumed post-Rolandic cortex (–25%) and other electrode sites. Nevertheless, in both figures it is apparent that the more symmetrical post-Rolandic region is approximately equal or greater in amplitude compared to the electrode site over presumed motor cortex. Another feature indicating the presence of separate symmetrical and asymmetrical components can be seen in figure 3; notice that the asymmetry of N1 differentially increases over the presumed motor cortex as movement onset is approached. These patterns are also reported by DEECKE and KORNHUBER [this volume]. Yet another indication of the dissociations which may be produced as a function of several variables may be seen when subject populations are broken down into subgroups of right- and left-handers. Notice in figure 4 that left-handed subjects seem to deviate from the patterns of asymmetry and amplitude, compared to right-handed subjects. The left-handed subjects seem to show less asymmetry over all electrode locations, and they have a symmetrical amplitude peak more isolated over presumed motor cortex (0%), compared to right-handed subjects. This pattern of results has also been reported by other workers [cf. DEECKE and KORNHUBER, this volume], although it was not interpreted by these authors as arising due to the superposition of slow potential components of separate functional origin.

Those interested in distinguishing these positive versus negative and symmetrical versus asymmetrical slow potential components should employ certain minimal techniques. First, at least 4 pairs of active electrode sites are needed to topographically isolate the various components. A

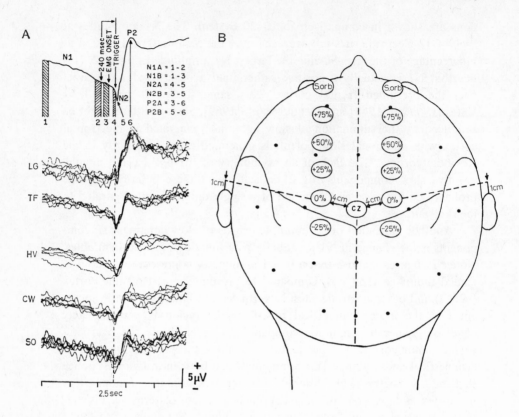

*Fig. 1. A* MPs over the presumed motor cortex are shown for each of 5 subjects (superimposed traces). The reliability of MP waveforms within subjects (superimposed sessions over days) and across subjects is evident even though each trace is an average of 64 responses for 4 subjects, 96 responses for SO. The vertical broken line indicates the photocell trigger onset. The top trace is the grand average of all these responses (N = 2, 112). The number 1–6 below the grand average indicate the data points between which wavelet measurements were derived as indicated at the upper right. *B* The 13 active electrode sites used to sample MP waveforms are compared to the 10–20 system (dots) and to the approximate location of the rolandic sulcus. Indifferent electrodes were placed either as balanced non-cephalic reference or linked superior-dorsal ear surface electrodes. Impedance of all electrodes was less than 5 kΩ.

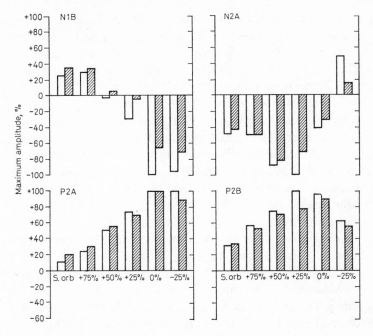

*Fig. 2.* Mean amplitudes (⁰/o of maximum) for three MP wavelets (N1, N2, P2) are measured over six pairs of electrodes. Positive amplitudes are indicated as histograms above the baseline; electrodes contralateral to movement are shown as unfilled bars, ipsilateral electrodes by oblique lines. Two types of measurement of the P2 wavelet are shown in order to indicate the effect of superposition of the N2 and P2 components with the P2B measurement.

frontal pair of electrodes (+75⁰/o sites, or Fp sites) is needed to record the 'N1' slow positivity and to monitor artifacts from eye movements. The diffuseness of symmetrical versus asymmetrical N1 components in left- and right-handed subjects can be assessed with electrode sites paired anterior to motor cortex (+25⁰/o sites, or F3, F4). The focus of asymmetrical N1 components is best observed over motor cortex (0⁰/o, or 1–2 cm anterior to C3, C4). The diffuseness and post-Rolandic dominance of symmetrical N1 components should be recorded with electrodes just posterior to the Central fissure (–25⁰/o, or between C3, C4 and P3, P4). The most important technical consideration remaining is that steps are taken to separate N1 components from the movement-adjacent components which overlap with N1 as movement onset is approached. Since some of these components are highly asymmetrical, while others are lacking asymmetry, N1 measurements may be affected by inclusion of these movement-adjacent components. Correspondingly, DEECKE et al. [1969] and GERBRANDT et al. [1973] recommend that N1 measurements be terminated 150 msec before onset of EMG. As EMG onset often occurs more than 150 msec in advance of the actual movement, movement-transduced triggers are likely to smear the movement-adjacent components over N1 at more than 150 msec before the mean EMG onset. At a minimum then, it is recommended that EMG onset be used to trigger MPs. Even here, the earliest responding principle effector should be monitored, and there is a danger that EMG recordings over a single muscle group may not represent the earliest EMG onset [GERBRANDT et al., 1973]. Movement-adjacent components could then be smeared over N1 even more than 150 msec in advance of such an EMG trigger. It is interesting then that certain movements, such as palmar flexions and fist contractions require several hundred trials of averaging to obtain reliable MP waveforms within subjects, and even here produce MP waveforms that are highly variable across subjects [GILDEN et al., 1966; DEECKE et al., 1969]. These variabilities may be due to the considerable complexity of muscle effectors involved in these movements. We have accordingly used simple index finger dorsal-extension as our abrupt voluntary movement [GERBRANDT et al., 1973]; reproducibility of the MP waveform within sessions (sets of 16 trial averages), across sessions, and across subjects may then be seen even with small numbers of trials (cf. fig. 1). SYNDULKO and LINDSLEY [this volume] also report clear results with this type of movement. Undetected rotations in the earliest responding msucle effectors may become even more likely with increased complexity of movements such as button-pressing and balloon-squeezing. As a result, the N1 and movement-adjacent components may again be blurred by superposition. For this reason, these movements should either be avoided in MP research, or multiple EMG monitoring should be used to guarantee that the earliest EMG activity is always used as the trigger for computer averaging.

Experimental manipulation of conditions which differentially affect the positive versus negative and symmetrical versus asymmetrical slow potential components may also be used to verify and control these multiple overlapping components. SYNDULKO and LINDSLEY [this volume] show that the frontal slow positive component is found in a combined

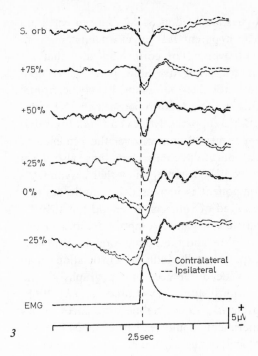

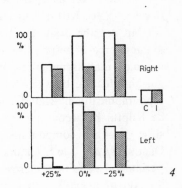

*Fig. 3.* MPs contralateral (solid traces) and ipsilateral (broken traces) to movement are shown for a single subject over 6 electrode locations. Each trace is an average of 64 responses. Integrated EMG activity is shown as the bottom pair of traces, and photocell onset (trigger for averages) is indicated by the vertical broken line. Changes in N1 asymmetry as a function of electrode location and timing before EMG onset, and two post-movement abrupt negativities superimposed on the P2 wavelet may be seen in this subject. The apparent reversal of the first post-movement abrupt negativity (+25%) to a positivity (–25%) may be superimposed on a poorly registered P1 wavelet.

*Fig. 4.* Mean amplitudes (% of maximum) for N1 wavelets measured from onset to 150 msec before EMG onset (N1A) are shown for three pairs of electrodes. Higher negative amplitudes are indicated as histograms above the baseline; electrodes contralateral to movement are shown as unfilled bars, ipsilateral electrodes as filled bars. The subject population shown in figure 2 is divided here into right- (top) and left- (bottom) handed subgroups of subjects (3 right-handed subjects, 2 left- handed subjects).

MP-CNV situation where visual cues are used as S1-S2, but not when auditory stimuli are substituted. The apparent lack of effect on the asymmetrical slow negative component over motor cortex indicates that the symmetrical positive and asymmetrical negative slow potential components can be dissociated. It should not then be assumed that the frontal slow positive component is a distinguishing feature between the N1 component of the MP and the CNV, which apparently lacks a frontal positivity only in certain conditions. Experimental control over the presence of symmetrical versus asymmetrical negative components has also been demonstrated. KUTAS and DONCHIN [this volume] show that a symmetrical but not the asymmetrical component is increased in amplitude as a greater force of responding is required of subjects. It should not then be assumed that asymmetries of the slow negative component are a distinguishing feature between N1 of the MP and the nonmotoric CNV. These topographically indicated and experimentally induced dissociations may be helpful in accounting for the wide differences in topography of the slow potential components in various studies [VAUGHAN et al., 1968; DEECKE et al., 1969; GERBRANDT et al., 1973]. Subtle differences in experimental conditions across experiments could lead to changes in positive versus negative and symmetrical versus asymmetrical slow potential components, and these changed topographies would lead to un necessary controversies about the functional origin of what has been thought to be a single N1 component.

### The Pre-Movement Positive Component

By the nomenclature used by VAUGHAN et al. [1968], the next MP wavelet after N1 is P1. Controversy exists as to whether this wavelet occurs before [VAUGHAN et al., 1968; DEECKE et al., 1969] or after [GERBRANDT et al., 1973] EMG onset, and whether its topography is consistent with an origin in motor [VAUGHAN et al., 1968] or parietal [DEECKE and KORNHUBER, this volume] cortex. What we interpret to be P1 occurred as a small positive deflection in only 1 of 5 subjects (cf. top subject in fig. 1), and just before movement and after EMG onset. It was best seen in recordings over presumed motor cortex. DEECKE and KORNHUBER [this volume] report that P1 (PMP by their nomenclature) is largest in amplitude and symmetrical over post-Rolandic cortex. They have previously reported that P1 is asymmetrically largest over the motor cortex ipsilateral to

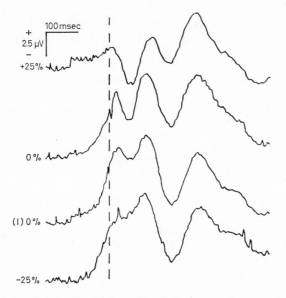

*Fig. 5.* MPs for subject LG (cf. fig. 1) are shown at 4 electrode sites when all trials were averaged in a single 8-hour session (1,024 trials), using an EMG trigger (vertical broken line). Notice the prominent P1 component before EMG onset, and the two post-movement abrupt negativities superimposed on a P2 wavelet.

movement [DEECKE *et al.*, 1969], but this apparently arose due to super-position of P1 with contralaterally asymmetrical movement-adjacent components (MP by their nomenclature). DEECKE and KORNHUBER [this volume] suggest that large numbers of trials in one experimental session, and an EMG trigger, are needed to maximize the P1 component relative to other components. Our results may then be consistent with this finding, but the limited amplitude of P1 under our experimental conditions may have obscured its earliest latency and correct topography.

In order to find whether a large number of trials and EMG triggering would resolve this controversy over the latency and origin of P1, the only subject showing the small P1 wavelet (fig. 1) moved his index finger every 10–20 sec for 8 h (1,024 successful trials) while EMG recordings were taken from a fine wire electrode placed intramuscularly into the principle effector for finger extension. In figure 5, it may be seen that P1 has not only grown substantially in amplitude relative to what we have previously termed the N2 component (fig. 1), but it is now occurring 60–90 msec be-fore EMG onset (dashed line). Also in agreement with DEECKE and

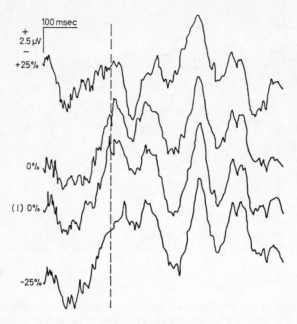

*Fig. 6.* MPs for subject LG are shown in an average of only 16 of the last successful trials in the 8-hour session referred to in figure 5. Notice that the P1 and other wavelets are also emergent within a few trials of averaging.

KORNHUBER [this volume] the P1 peak amplitude is now largest over presumed post-Rolandic cortex. These data, however, do not indicate that large numbers of trials need be averaged to see P1. In figure 6, notice that an average of only 16 trials taken from the end of the 8-hour session indicates that P1 is emerging. Indeed, in the last half of the 8-hour session, P1 is often apparent in the raw EEG records. These results were not found within the first 128 trials of this session. The large size of P1 relative to other wavelets in the late part of a long session may provide a clue as to how experimental control over P1 may be gained in a small number of trials. Could it be that subjects attempt to nullify the boredom of extended trials and redundant movements by developing ancillary routines which are synchronized to movements? We have noted, for example, that some subjects admit to subvocalizing expressions such as 'now' or to counting their movements. Future research should concentrate on the types of experimental variables which enhance and eliminate the P1 component. These may or may not be consistent with a mere volitional decision to move [cf. DEECKE and KORNHUBER, this volume].

## Pre- and Post-Movement Negative Components

The most controversial issue which has arisen over the MP concerns the timing and topography of the second negative wavelet apparent in monopolar records (N2). We have found [GERBRANDT et al., 1973] that N2 is largest over the cortex anterior to motor cortex (cf. fig. 2, 3) and follows EMG onset whether or not MP averages are triggered by EMG onset (fig. 5). The occurrence of N2 about 20–50 msec after EMG onset and its similarity in scalp distribution to the SEP (cf. fig. 3, 7) has led us to the conclusion that it arises due to reafference from movement. These results and conclusions are in apparent conflict with those of VAUGHAN et al. [1968] and DEECKE et al. [1969]. The latter but not the former investigators report that N2 (MP by their nomenclature) is largest over the motor cortex. Both groups find N2 to precede rather than follow EMG onset.

It now seems that this controversy can be resolved. The finding (fig. 5) that the temporal relationship to EMG onset and the N2 scalp distribution did not change when averages were formed using an EMG trigger and large numbers of trials indicates that our prior results have not arisen because of these technical considerations. A remaining possibility is that we have explicitly measured an abrupt negative component which is not the N2 component referred to by other MP investigators. An abrupt negative wavelet, which is largest in front of motor cortex and has its peak at about the same time after EMG onset as we have found, may be seen in the published monopolar records of other workers (fig. 2, 3, 5) [VAUGHAN et al., 1968; DEECKE et al., 1969]. Its topography and relationship to EMG onset are not examined in these papers. Instead, DEECKE et al. [1969] measure the second negative component (N2) in bipolar derivations (contralateral minus ipsilateral). In fact, they note that the superposition of the P1 component with N2 (MP by their terminology) obscures N2 in monopolar recordings; in monopolar records, N2 is inferred from the smaller P1 contralateral to movement. This depression of the monopolar P1 amplitude over the contralateral motor cortex can be seen before the onset of EMG, and before what we have previously termed N2 (fig. 6). It seems then, that the second negativity which appears before the onset of EMG when bipolar derivations are used [DEECKE et al., 1969] is probably not due to the same negative component which arises after EMG onset in our monopolar records. Until a commonly agreed upon nomenclature is devised, we will call the MP wavelet of DEECKE et al. [1969] 'N2', and the post-EMG negativity of GERBRANDT et al. [1973] 'N3'.

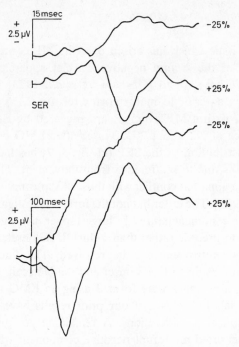

*Fig. 7.* The similarities of waveform and topographic distribution are shown for the early wavelets of an SER (top pair of traces) and the first post-movement abrupt negativity of the MP (bottom pair of traces). Both are negative going in front of the Rolandic sulcus (+25% site), and appear to reverse in polarity posterior to the Rolandic sulcus (−25% site). Both are averages of 128 trials. The MP waveforms are shown after the first two of a series of incrementing EMG points indicating EMG onset (vertical bars).

Certain technical and experimental conditions should be used in order to differentiate these movement-adjacent MP components. The 4 pairs of electrodes needed to dissociate the various slow MP components are also needed to differentiate these movement-adjacent components. The distribution of P1 can be followed monopolarly from electrodes anterior to motor cortex (near +25%) to its peak over post-Rolandic cortex (near −25%). Bipolar derivations over the same electrode pairs (contralateral-ipsilateral) are needed to show the focus over motor cortex of the pre-movement negative component (N2) of DEECKE et al. [1969]. As noted above, bipolar derivations should be used to eliminate the superposition of P1 components in N2 measurements. Since the N1 component gains in asymmetry as EMG onset is approached, and since it has a topography similar to N2, care should also be taken to differentiate N2 from superpositions with the tail of N1. Owing to their similarities in topography, this can be done only if experimental conditions are found which will differentially enhance either component relative to the other. In left-handed subjects, for example, N1 can be made more asymmetrical by use of the non-dominant hand [KUTAS and DONCHIN, this volume]. If future research shows that N1 asymmetry generally grows while N2 asymmetry is constant, then the assumption that the asymmetrical N1 and N2 components are of separate functional origin [DEECKE and KORNHUBER, this volume] would be supported. The same 4 pairs of electrodes are also needed to record the post-movement abrupt negative component (N3) of GERBRANDT et al. [1973]. The peak amplitude of N3 is best seen anterior to motor cortex (near $+25^0/_0$). Its apparent reversal is seen over post-Rolandic cortex (near $-25^0/_0$). Bipolar derivations (contralateral-ipsilateral) here should help to resolve the apparent reversal of N3 without the superposition of P1. Subtraction of the post-Rolandic bipolar derivation from the $+25^0/_0$ bipolar derivation should reveal the N3 component across the Rolandic line without superposition from either N1 or P1. Finally, whereas N2 and N3 components can probably be experimentally dissociated from N1 and P2 components, dissociations of N2 and N3 amplitudes should be difficult to produce in neurologically normal persons. N2 onset occurs about 50 msec before movement, allowing little influence from psychological variables. N3 occurs within 50 msec after EMG onset, and is also likely to be immune from psychological variables. Feedback (N3) without command (N2) can be simulated with passive movement of the finger; it is interesting therefore that an abrupt negative wavelet distributed similar to N3 is found shortly after passive movement of the finger [KORNHUBER and DEECKE, 1965].

## Post-Movement Components

It has been assumed that there is only one post-movement MP component, namely P2 [VAUGHAN et al., 1968]. As noted above, an abrupt negative wavelet (N3) should be recognized as occurring within 50 msec after EMG onset. Furthermore, a second negative wavelet (N4) often appears about 120–180 msec after EMG onset, and is largest over the post-Rolandic region (fig. 3, 5). Its smaller size at pre-Rolandic sites, and its superposition there with relatively larger MP components (P1, N3 and

P2) may result in its being seen there (fig. 1) as a notch on the transition from N3 to P2. Little is known about the functional origin or techniques needed to record N4. The movements used to induce it should be very abrupt in onset, and sustained in order to eliminate complications of MP waveforms due to multiple movements. The fact that it is a relatively fast wavelet riding on the slower P2 wavelet, suggests that faster time constants could be used to bring it out relative to P2. Its relationship to the peak of EMG activity, suggests that it may be related either to the termination of movement onset, or to the change from a movement to a sustained response. Its similarity in distribution to the P1 component (fig. 3, 5) suggests that N4 could be the return of the P1 component to baseline. Experimentally induced dissociations of the P1 and N4 components are therefore needed.

The final component to be discussed here is the P2 component (fig. 1). It was originally thought to be contralaterally asymmetrical and largest in amplitude over the motor cortex [VAUGHAN et al., 1968]. GERBRANDT et al. [1973] subsequently showed that such asymmetries and anteriorly shifted amplitude peaks can result from the inclusion of the superposed N3 component in the measurements of P2 (cf. P2A versus P2B measures in fig. 1 and 2). P2 onset should probably be measured prior to EMG onset; then it has little or no symmetry, and is largest over post-Rolandic cortex. Even here, there is a danger that its distribution is being affected by superposition with N1 components. Experimentally induced dissociations between P2 and all other components should then be attempted. Unfortunately, there is yet little basis for suggesting what these conditions might be. If P2 is a movement-homolog of the exteroceptive 'uncertainty wave' of SUTTON et al. [1967], then it may be that P2 itself results from multiple overlapping late positive components, which must be dissected from each other in topography by numerous experimental conditions [cf. RITTER et al., this series].

## Conclusions

It appears from the complexities of MP waveforms at several sites that there may be at least 8 components in the usual MP waveform. Considerable overlap exists in the timing and distributions of each of these components. The main implication of these possible superpositions of multiple MP components is that the question is raised as to how singular functional interpretations can be validly ascribed to wavelets which are composed of multiple MP components, when experimentally induced dissociations from other components have not been demonstrated in humans. Largely on the basis of topographic appearance, the entire waveform, for example, was thought to be motoric in functional origin [VAUGHAN *et al.*, 1968]. Other investigators have questioned this interpretation on the basis that the topographies they find indicate only one [DEECKE *et al.*, 1969] or no [GERBRANDT *et al.*, 1973] MP components are motoric in origin. These discrepancies in findings are discussed above as arising because experimenters vary in the extent to which they increase the superposition of MP components with each other by the measurements they have used, by how the averages are triggered, by the choice of movement and sampling of EMG onset, by the number of trials averaged in a session, and by the over-reliance on topographic observations and timing relationships to EMG onset to give clues as to the functional origin of MP wavelets.

The resolution of each MP component in isolation from other MP components seems to be an unrealized but necessary goal, before agreement can be reached on the functional origins of each MP component. Two directions in future MP research are likely to be helpful in this regard. First, techniques more appropriate than mapping of scalp potential gradients should be used to infer the anatomical generators of MP components. Detailed laminar analysis of the sort reported on the origin of SEP components [GOFF *et al.*, this series] should be helpful. Alternatively, techniques should be developed for mapping the current densities of MP components over the scalp [PERL and CASBY, 1954], and in depth [FREEMAN and STONE, 1969], as these current waveforms should be more highly localized than potential gradients. Second, experimental conditions must be identified which can dissociate each MP component from all others. This will help to resolve the topography of each component. Also, regardless of the topographic origin and relationship to EMG onset, the functional origin of MP components are best determined by which experimental variables control them. Correspondingly, the MP nomenclature should not be used as an implicit, premature statement of the functional origin of the MP waveform. The suggestion here is that the MP waveform be referred to as *movement potential* waveform and not a *motor potential*. The reference to MP wavelets as *the readiness potential, the motor potential*, etc., should also be avoided as they are implicit singular functional interpretations.

## References

DEECKE, L.; SCHEID, P., and KORNHUBER, H. H.: Distribution of readiness potential, pre-motion positivity, and motor potential of the human cerebral cortex preceding voluntary finger movements. Expl Brain Res. 7: 158–168 (1969).

FREEMAN, V. A. and STONE, J.: A technique for current density analysis of field potentials and its application to the frog cerebellum; in LLINAS Neurobiology of cerebellar evolution and development (Am. Medical Ass., Chicago 1969).

GERBRANDT, L. K.; GOFF, W. R., and SMITH, D. B.: Distribution of the human average movement potential. Electroenceph. clin. Neurophysiol. 34: 461–474 (1973).

GILDEN, L.; VAUGHAN, H. G., jr., and COSTA, L. D.: Summated human EEG potentials with voluntary movement. Electroenceph. clin. Neurophysiol. 20: 433–438 (1966).

KORNHUBER, H. H. und DEECKE, L.: Hirnpotentialänderungen bei Willkürbewegungen und passiven Bewegungen des Menschen: Bereitschaftspotential und reafferente Potentiale. Pflügers Arch. ges. Physiol. 284: 1–17 (1965).

PERL, E. R. and CASBY, J. V.: Localization of cerebral electrical activity: the acoustic cortex of cat. J. Neurophysiol. 17: 429–442 (1954).

SUTTON, S.; TUETING, P.; ZUBIN, J., and JOHN, E. R.: Information delivery and the sensory evoked potential. Science 155: 1436–1439 (1967).

VAUGHAN, H. G., jr.; COSTA, L. D., and RITTER, W.: Topography of the human motor potential. Electroenceph. clin. Neurophysiol. 25: 1–10 (1968).

Dr. L. K. GERBRANDT, Department of Psychology, California State University, Northridge, CA 91324 (USA)

Attention, Voluntary Contraction and Event-Related Cerebral Potentials.
Prog. clin. Neurophysiol., vol. 1, Ed. J. E. DESMEDT, pp. 189–210 (Karger, Basel 1977)

# The Effect of Handedness, of Responding Hand, and of Response Force on the Contralateral Dominance of the Readiness Potential

MARTA KUTAS and EMANUEL DONCHIN

Cognitive Psychophysiology Laboratory, Department of Psychology,
University of Illinois at Champaign, Champaign, Ill.

## Preliminary Note on Nomenclature

In this paper we will identify movement-related potentials with labels proposed by VAUGHAN et al. [1968]. While this system is not consistent with the recommendations of the Methodology Committee (this volume) in that the components will be identified ordinally, we feel that there will be no ambiguity in our usage when applied to movement-related potentials. The nomenclature recommended by the Methodology Committee is appropriate for naming potential peaks, either positive or negative, but not for naming slopes, for which latency cannot be meaningfully specified. Some writers refer to the components in question with labels like 'readiness potentials' (RP), 'reafferent potentials', etc. Such labels which of course imply a certain theoretical position concerning the origin and functional significance of the potentials should be avoided. In this report, therefore, the term RP is used to refer to a theoretical process underlying pre-response negativity which we shall call $N_1$. Whether $N_1$ is a manifestation of a RP is the central issue of our study.

## Introduction

It has been reliably established that, during the foreperiod of a reaction time task, a slow negative cerebral potential develops which peaks just before the presentation of the imperative stimulus whereupon it gives place to a rapidly changing, positive-going cortical potential. WALTER [1964] labelled this negative shift, the contingent negative variation (CNV). The CNV has been reported to reflect psychological constructs such as expectancy [WALTER *et al.*, 1964], conation [Low *et al.*, 1966], motivation [IRWIN *et al.*, 1966; REBERT *et al.*, 1967], and attention [MCCALLUM, 1969; WEINBERG, 1973]. While the CNV is currently assumed to be primarily a manifestation of cognitive/perceptual activity, there is no consensus on its functional significance. The interpretation of the CNV has been complicated when KORNHUBER and DEECKE [1965] as well as VAUGHAN and co-workers [GILDEN *et al.*, 1966; VAUGHAN *et al.*, 1968; VAUGHAN, 1969] reported that self-paced voluntary activity was also preceded by a slow cerebral potential having both a slow pre-response negative component and post-response positivity. The positive post-response potential had originally been described by BATES [1951] and DONCHIN and LINDSLEY [1966], but the pre-response potentials had not been previously reported. These movement-related potentials have been differentiated into four components: (1) a ramp-shaped negative potential which begins to develop 800–1000 msec prior to the movement ($N_1$); (2) a rapid acceleration at the end of $N_1$ ($N_2$); (3) a rapid, small amplitude positive wave ($P_1$) reported to occur between $N_1$ and $N_2$, and (4) a large positive wave ($P_2$) which follows $N_2$. Whereas GILDEN *et al.* [1966] referred to this entire complex as 'motor potentials', implying that they are indicators of '... physiological correlates of preparatory motor sets and readiness for movement', DEECKE *et al.* [1969] consider only the $P_1$ and $N_2$ components to be 'motor' potentials and consider $N_1$ a 'Bereitschaft' or 'readiness' potential (RP), thus pointing to some similarity between the CNV and the RP. Other investigators have also suggested that the CNV and $N_1$ may be related. Some have said the CNV might be a RP [GILDEN *et al.*, 1966; Low *et al.*, 1966], others that the RP might be a CNV [DEECKE *et al.*, 1969; COHEN, 1969]. VAUGHAN viewed the CNV as an index of a response-related readiness associated with control processes in the pyramidal system rather than with global mobilization in anticipation of some external stimulus. More recent formulations proposed that $N_1$ may be a sum of several independent event-related slow potentials [HILL-YARD, 1973] and the nature of the $N_1$-CNV relation remains unclear.

In most CNV studies, subjects were to respond to the imperative stimulus (S2), with a movement (e.g. a button press). In fact, the close association of the CNV with the subject's intention to make a response contingent on S2 was emphasized by WALTER and led him to postulate a response-priming function for processes underlying the CNV. However, the slow cortical negativity is not dependent upon the execution of a motor response after the imperative stimulus [COHEN and WALTER, 1966; Low et al., 1966; DONCHIN et al., 1972, 1973]. Yet, while CNVs can be elicited in the absence of a motor response, the execution of a response after S2 increases the amplitude of the CNV [WALTER, 1964; IRWIN et al., 1966; LOW et al., 1966; PETERS et al., 1970]. IRWIN et al. [1966] have pointed out that the enhancement of CNV magnitude by a subsequent motor response is of the same order (10–15 $\mu$V) as the $N_1$ produced prior to a voluntary movement. Further, this slow surface negativity is significantly larger when a large amount of force, or muscular effort, is required as the response to S2 [LOW and MCSHERRY, 1968; REBERT et al., 1967].

Another attempt at the dissection of the motor from the non-motor aspects of pre-response potentials has been made by studying the scalp distribution of the potentials. The CNV's distribution is reportedly symmetric around a peak at the vertex, somewhat smaller in the frontal areas and smallest in the posterior region [LOW et al., 1966]. The cortical distribution of $N_1$ depends according to VAUGHAN et al. [1968] on the responding limb and is somatotopically related to the muscles involved in the movement. While these data suggest that $N_1$ and CNV are distinct, there are reports [OTTO and LEIFER, 1973; SYNDULKO and LINDSLEY, this volume] that in a forewarned unimanual task the pre-response negativity is greater over the sensorimotor area contralateral to the responding hand. Of course, an asymmetric distribution of the potential is most consistent with the notion that it reflects activity of the motor cortex associated with preparation for movement.

The present study was an attempt to determine the degree to which parameters of the motor response determine the waveform, amplitude, and hemispheric distribution of the $N_1$ component. The $N_1$ features were chosen for study because there is some question as to whether the later components of the motor potential occur before or after the motor response [cf. DEECKE and KORNHUBER, this volume; RITTER et al., this series]. The response variables manipulated were response force and the responding hand. Since the motor cortex is directly involved in the control of muscle force [EVARTS, 1967], it could be expected that some cerebral motor preparation specific to one hand would be maximal over the contralateral pre-rolandic area. This problem cannot yet be clarified from published data and possible differences related to the subject's handedness should also be considered. The present experiment was designed to determine the distribution of $N_1$ over the motor areas when both left and right- handed subjects responded with either hand, using three different force levels to respond.

## Method

Subjects: Eleven University students (7 right-handed and 4 left-handed) were paid for participating in the experiment. Handedness was determined by self-report, subsequently verified by the Edinburgh Inventory [OLDFIELD, 1971].

Recording procedures: Beckman biopotential electrodes (No. 6509) filled with Beckman electrode paste were secured to the subject's scalp with collodion at $C_z$, $C_4$, and $C_3$ and were referred to a linked mastoid electrode. Electrode impedance, measured with a Grass E-Z-M impedance meter, did not exceed 10 kΩ. Right supraorbital and canthal electrodes (fastened with adhesive collars) were used to record the electrooculogram (EOG). The electromyogram (EMG) was recorded from the responding arm, one electrode at a third of the distance from the lateral humeral epicondyle to the styloid process of the ulna and the other approximately 1.5–2 inches in the distal direction along the same line. Signals were amplified with Brush amplifiers (No. 13-4218–00) with bandwidth setting of 0.1–30 Hz (6 dB/octave roll-off, i.e. the time constant was 1.51 sec). EMG activity was recorded by means of a Grass Model 7P3 preamplifier and integrator combination (1/2 amplitude low frequency = 0.3, time constant = 0.02). Data were recorded on a Hewlett-Packard 3955 FM tape recorder at $1^7/_8$ ips and averaged off-line with either a PDP/8E or an IBM 1800. All trials in which detectable, gross eye movements occurred were not used in averaging. Trials were included if the sum of squares of digitized EOG voltages did not exceed a criterion value.

Procedure: The subject sat in a comfortable chair inside of an electrically shielded, darkened room fixating a dim square displayed continuously in a scope. Subjects were instructed to rapidly squeeze a Dynamometer constructed by attaching a Daytronic model 152A, LDVT force transducer to a grip-handle. The displacement of the dynamometer was 0.25 mm at all applied force levels. We determined for each subject a maximal force level for each hand by asking the subject to rapidly squeeze the dynamometer several times as hard as he could. The force levels the subjects generated during test series were defined as 0.25, 0.50, and 0.75 of their maximal force. The actual force levels used were 0.25 = 5 kg, 0.5 = 10 kg, and 0.75 = 15 kg for the non-dominant hand, and 0.25 = 7 kg, 0.5 = 12.5 kg, and 0.75 = 20 kg (± 1 kg) for the dominant hand.

To provide the subjects with feedback concerning their emitted force, a transilluminated circle was superimposed on the fixation square. Subjects were told to find the squeeze force level that would just extinguish the circle. The circle, once extinguished, was reilluminated after 1 sec. The electronics made it possible to arrange the extinction of the stimulus at any preset force level. Subjects were cautioned against overpressing. Within each session there were two separate runs. In the first, the subjects generated a series of 50–100 similar squeezes, each extinguishing the feedback circle for a short period. In the second run, subjects were instructed to continue squeezing the dynamometer at the same level that previously extinguished the light, without the visual feedback. Except for two test cases, in any one session, voluntary movements were performed using one hand only at each of the three force levels, and always in the order 0.25, 0.50, and 0.75. Each subject participated in a minimum of six sessions, three with each hand. The order of hand usage was counterbalanced across different subjects.

## Results

*Pattern of motor responses of the subjects.* The output of the dyna-mometer served to time-lock the averaging of ERPs recorded at $C_3$ and $C_4$ scalp locations and it was continuously recorded, along with the EMG of forearm flexors. Analysis of these data served to assess the relationship between the nominal force requested in the instructions and the actual force produced. Figure 1A presents the force traces for a series of succes-sive trials at one nominal force. The course of the traces is reasonably un-iform from onset to peak, but is variable after dynamometer release. A study of confidence limits of average force curves per series showed this to be the common pattern. In the early part of a session, subjects squeezed the dynamometer at rather irregular intervals, but they gradual-ly shifted to a more regular squeezing rate; interspersed with rest periods. The minimum interval was 3 sec and the maximum 8 sec (fig. 1B). Figure 2 presents the means and SD for peak force measurements in right- and left-handed subjects, in all experimental conditions. An analysis of the variance of these data showed that: (a) the actual peak force is a mono-tonically increasing function of the nominal force levels, with the distribu-tions of actual force exhibiting only minimal overlap; (b) the mean peak values are consistently smaller for the non-dominant hand, and (c) in the condition without feedback, the response force always exceeds that gener-ated during the corresponding feedback condition. These data suggest that on the whole the subjects behaved as instructed.

*Fig. 1. A* Superposition of traces of movement force obtained in a series of successive trials at one nominal force level in one subject. *B* The force responses shown in *A* are displayed on a slower time base to indicate the variability of the in-tervals between successive trials and of the force amplitude. The upper traces are the trigger pulses used to mark events, the lower traces represent the output of the force transducer. The horizontal sweep represents 800 msec in *A* and 20 sec in *B*.

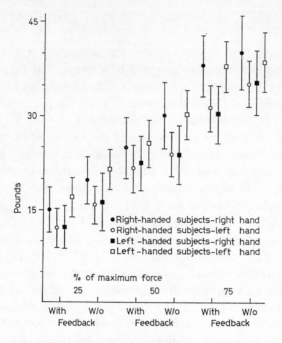

*Fig. 2.* The means and standard deviations of the peak mean force measurements plotted as a function of the subjects' handedness and the responding hand in all experimental conditions.

*Waveform of average ERP.* There was a considerable similarity between the waveforms recorded from $C_3$ and $C_4$ scalp electrodes in all subjects. The right-handed subjects showed substantially less variability (fig. 3, 4). In view of this consistency between subjects, we used in subsequent figures the grand ('over-subject') averages for right-handed and left-handed subjects, respectively (fig. 5), thus comparing ERPs from $C_3$ (solid line) and $C_4$ (dashed line) locations when responding with either the right or the left hand, at the three chosen levels of squeeze force. The average integrated EMG (dashed line) and force output (solid line) are presented below the ERP records in figure 5.

In agreement with previously published data, a slow negativity developed prior to movement ($N_1$), and this accelerated at about the time of the movement ($N_2$) and was followed by a positive-going wave ($P_2$). The $P_1$ component, called pre-motion positivity by DEECKE and KORNHUBER [cf. this volume], was difficult to identify in our records.

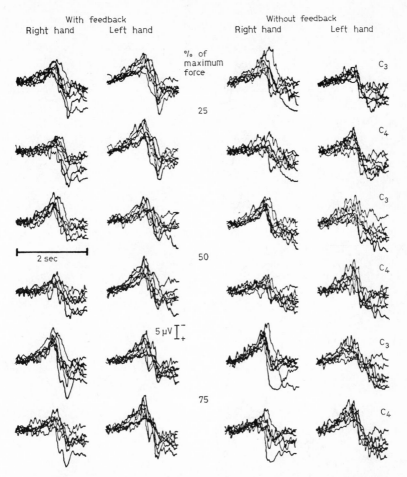

*Fig. 3.* Superposition of event-related potentials (ERPs) obtained from each of the 7 right-handed subjects at the C₃ and C₄ electrodes, for each responding hand at each force level for each feedback condition. Avarages were obtained over all subjects after the elimination of trials in which the EEG was contaminated by EOG activity. Number of trials per ERP ranges between 100 and 400.

When right-handed subjects perform a self-paced voluntary movement, the premotion negativity ($N_1$) is consistently larger over the sensorimotor location contralateral to the hand used. This asymmetry is evident (in some cases) as early as 500 msec before the initiation of the movement, as defined by EMG onset. The hemispheric difference in $N_1$ is smaller for left-hand responses. Contralateral dominance is apparent

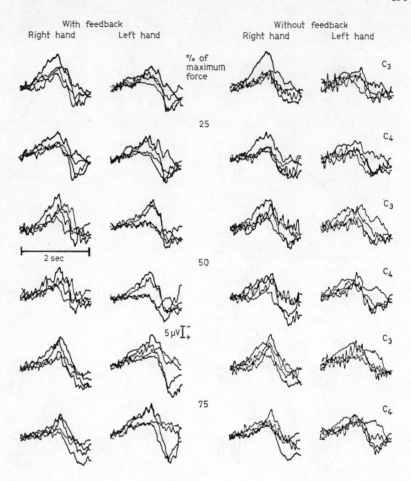

*Fig. 4.* Superposition of ERPs obtained from each of the 4 left-handed subjects at the $C_3$ and $C_4$ locations, for each responding hand at each force level and feedback condition.

(though reduced) in the left-handed subjects when they respond with their right hand (fig. 5). Thus, $N_1$ is maximal over the hemisphere contralateral to the responding hand for right hand responses, independent of subject handedness. This is *not* the case for left hand responses. While left-handed subjects show contralateral dominance when using their right hand, they generally show bilaterally symmetric waveforms when responding with their left hand. Occasionally, a left-handed subject would show a slight degree of contralateral dominance preceding left-hand squeezes.

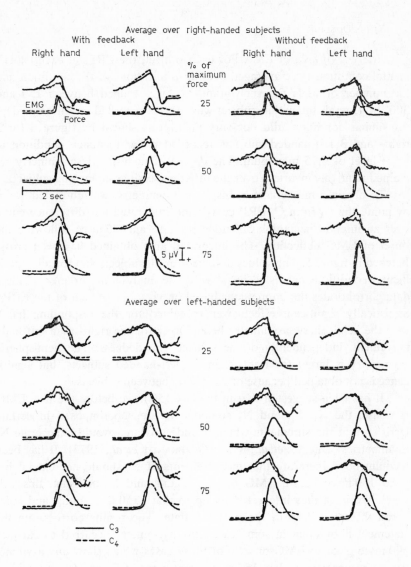

*Fig. 5.* A comparison of ERPs recorded at electrodes placed at left central ($C_3$, solid line) and right central ($C_4$, dashed line) loci during voluntary squeezes. Under each pair of superimposed ERPs, we plot the integrated EMG (dashed line) and the output of the force transducer (solid line) averaged over the same trials over which the ERP was averaged. Comparisons are presented as a function of the subject's handedness (right vs left), nominal force output (25, 50, and 75% of subject's maximal force), responding hand (right vs left) and feedback (with vs without). Number of trials per ERP ranges between 600 and 1,050. The cross-hatched areas in two of the comparison illustrate the areas measured for the purpose of the quantitative data analysis.

*Analysis of area of ERP.* For each subject, the ERPs at each experimental condition were averaged over all replications of the condition and the number of trials per such grand averages ranged between 150 and 300. In general, the within-subject wave forms recorded on different days for similar conditions did not vary greatly, as shown by figure 6 for 3 right- and 3 left-handed subjects recorded under feedback condition at force level of 0.75 maximum. The degree of hemispheric asymmetry remained relatively invariant over the different sessions in any one subject.

To obtain a measure of hemispheric asymmetry, we subtracted, point by point, the $C_3$ from $C_4$ ERP curves and integrated this difference curve over an interval beginning 500 msec prior to and 25 msec following the onset of EMG deflection. The integrated area obtained has been cross-hatched in figure 5. The values obtained for all subjects and for all experimental conditions are listed in table I. The analysis of variance of these data corroborates the impressions based on visual inspection of the ERPs. Statistically significant effects were obtained for the responding hand, with the hemispheric asymmetry being larger for the right- than left-hand movement, independently of the subjects' handedness. The hemispheric asymmetry is larger for right- than for left-handed subjects, but significance is not obtained because of variability between subjects.

It has been suggested that in the last 150 msec before the first EMG response, the $N_1$, $P_1$, and $N_2$ components are superimposed in certain leads so that measurements which include this area would exaggerate $N_1$ asymmetries [DEECKE et al., 1969; GERBRANDT et al., 1973]. It has been recommended therefore that measurements of $N_1$ should not extend beyond 150 msec before EMG onset [DEECKE and KORNHUBER, this volume]. We have thus integrated $N_1$ up to that −150 msec point and compared these results with the previous data. The results corroborate the statement above that in some cases, the asymmetry occurred as early as 500 msec prior to EMG onset. For those cases which show *any* asymmetry, the asymmetry at the −150 msec point between $C_3$ and $C_4$ was evident in 83% of the right-handed subjects using their right hand, in 76% of the same subjects using their left hand, in 70% of the left-handed subjects using their right hand, and in 90% of the left-handed subjects using their left hand.

The ERP analysis also indicated that response force had no statistically significant effect on the hemispheric asymmetry. An analysis of the effect of the response force on the area under the ERP recorded at vertex ($C_z$), at $C_3$ and at $C_4$ for the 500 msec preceding and the 25 msec follow-

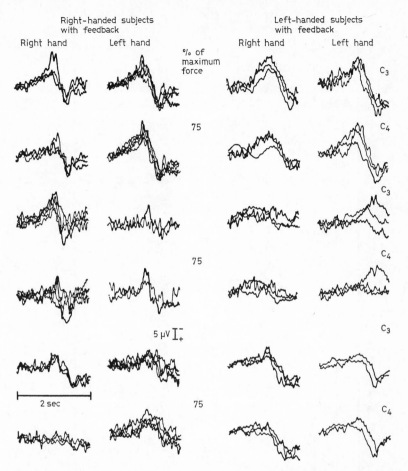

*Fig. 6.* Superposition of ERPs recorded at $C_3$ and $C_4$ locations during voluntary squeezes with the 75% nominal force and with feedback conditions. Each set
of comparisons for right- and left-hand response conditions are made with data recorded from one subject at various recording sessions (i.e. different days). Records
are provided for 3 right-handed and 3 left-handed subjects.

ing EMG onset showed that the force had a slight effect at all electrode
sites. However, there was no significant force $\times$ electrode interaction and
the degree of contralateral dominance seemed independent of the force
produced.

The force output and the EMG were quite similar in their initial segments. In general, the EMG onset preceded that of force by 50–80 msec.
The EMG onset always followed the appearance of asymmetry of $N_1$, but

*Table I.* Areas of pre-response negativity in difference curves ($C_4$–$C_3$)

| | | Right-handed subjects | | | | | | | Left-handed subjects | | | |
|---|---|---|---|---|---|---|---|---|---|---|---|---|
| | | J.E. | C.G. | J.H. | D.L. | D.T. | T.T. | M.C. | T.E. | R.S. | C.T. | G.W. |
| **Right hand** | | | | | | | | | | | | |
| 25% | w | 696 | 1,691 | 3,492 | –417 | 2,197 | 5,518 | 1,516 | 3,077 | 3,529 | 1,143 | 108 |
| | w/o | 2,937 | 2,588 | 2,448 | 2,328 | 3,603 | 5,638 | 2,453 | 3,701 | 464 | 2,641 | 250 |
| 50% | w | 2,744 | 1,688 | 2,628 | –1,002 | 2,990 | 1,602 | 3,489 | 1,244 | 3,055 | 3,843 | 952 |
| | w/o | 1,135 | 4,497 | 14,879 | 1,289 | 2,958 | 3,005 | 3,626 | 2,352 | 1,226 | 629 | 495 |
| 75% | w | 3,296 | 1,038 | 2,685 | 2,141 | 3,919 | 2,200 | 1,792 | 2,826 | 1,829 | 2,083 | –838 |
| | w/o | 5,396 | 4,373 | 2,672 | 2,341 | 3,949 | 5,332 | 1,317 | 2,464 | 1,463 | 2,348 | –295 |
| **Left hand** | | | | | | | | | | | | |
| 25% | w | –640 | 958 | 192 | –2,226 | –1,677 | –1,603 | 843 | –804 | –1,785 | –2,675 | 879 |
| | w/o | 106 | –112 | 4,134 | –2,456 | –1,755 | –490 | –1,643 | –85 | –586 | –1,483 | –1,548 |
| 50% | w | –1,292 | –1,168 | –2,755 | –1,026 | –2,218 | –2,565 | –11 | –293 | –807 | –1,639 | –1,206 |
| | w/o | –2,615 | 665 | 613 | 1,339 | –1,333 | –37 | –1,608 | 196 | –1,892 | –2,320 | 1,880 |
| 75% | w | –621 | 233 | –1,172 | –3,361 | –1,713 | –2,622 | 814 | 503 | –491 | –2,199 | –354 |
| | w/o | –2,259 | 1,310 | –4,493 | –2,345 | –1,482 | –4,105 | –169 | 454 | –1,635 | 948 | –645 |

it occurred either before, during, or after the peak negativity (called $N_2$), depending unsystematically on subject and condition. On the whole and to the extent that $P_1$ can be identified in our records, it appears that $P_1$ (and also $N_2$) would coincide with or follow the movement onset, peaking at or slightly before the EMG peak.

*Post-movement potentials.* The other major component of the motor potential, $P_2$, was recorded consistently in all subjects as a relatively large and complex positive-negative wave occurring after the movement; a marked difference in the sharpness of the positive peak can be observed for data obtained during the with- and without feedback conditions. $P_2$ peaks on the average 290–340 msec after the feedback stimulus in the feedback condition, whereas it is usually broader and flatter in the without feedback condition. This finding is again most consistent in the right-handed subjects.

*Principal component analysis.* The above analyses were based on either visual inspection or on the somewhat arbitrarily chosen area measure for each ERP record. As there has been some question as to the proper measure of $N_1$ independent from $N_2$ and of $P_2$ as well, we performed a factor analysis on the actual evoked response waveforms in the manner discussed by DONCHIN [1966]. All the ERPs were condensed to arrays of 50 points (40 msec per point). The principal axes of the entire $50 \times 132$ matrix were obtained, and a varimax rotation performed. In figure 7B, we plot the factor loadings of the five principal axes (accounting for 92.6% of the variance). The waveform averaged over all 132 ERPs is also plotted, for reference, in fig. 7A. The first factor (which accounted for 31% of the variance) appears heavily loaded on variables associated with the overall waveform. The second factor (25%) clearly represents points associated with the baseline, the third (19%) with $N_1$, the fourth (13%) with the transition points from $N_2$ to $P_2$, and the fifth (5.8%) primarily with $P_2$.

The factor scores obtained by applying the loadings for each of the 50 variables to the standardized matrix of raw data used in producing the factors were then subjected to an analysis of variance. The analysis was performed on all of the factor scores associated with each of the factors for each of the 132 evoked responses obtained from the eleven subjects for the six experimental conditions. Much of the variance is accounted for by the waveform factor which is significantly affected by the electrode position ($C_3$, $C_4$ and $C_z$) and various electrode interactions (electrode $\times$ responding hand and electrode $\times$ force). On the whole, these analyses simply confirm the results reported above.

*Table II.* Anova summary table of factor scores with dependent variable (factor 5 or component P₂)

| Source | d.f. | SS | MS | MS error | f | p |
|---|---|---|---|---|---|---|
| Handedness (A) | 1/9 | 4.5678 | 4.5678 | F | 0.36 | 0.55892 |
| Responding hand (B) | 1/9 | 1.6909 | 1.6909 | B × F | 0.51 | 0.49168 |
| Force (C) | 2/18 | 0.6938 | 0.3469 | C × F | 0.4979 | 0.61592 |
| Feedback (D) | 1/9 | 49.3711 | 49.3711 | D × F | 8.24 | 0.01845 |
| Electrode (E) | 2/18 | 0.8472 | 0.4236 | E × F | 0.95 | 0.40367 |
| Handedness × responding hand | 1/9 | 0.0680 | 0.0680 | B × F | 0.01 | 0.89487 |
| Handedness × force | 2/18 | 1.8438 | 0.9219 | C × F | 1.32 | 0.29101 |
| Handeduess × feedback | 1/9 | 16.8839 | 16.8839 | D × F | 2.81 | 0.12747 |
| Handedness- × electrode | 2/18 | 0.8040 | 0.4020 | E × F | 0.90 | 0.42188 |
| Responding hand × force | 2/18 | 4.5986 | 2.2993 | B × C × F | 2.29 | 0.12924 |
| Responding hand × feedback | 1/9 | 1.3203 | 1.3203 | B × D × F | 1.28 | 0.28596 |
| Responding hand × electrode positions | 2/18 | 2.1775 | 1.0887 | B × E × F | 3.41 | 0.05524 |
| Force × feedback | 2/18 | 1.1033 | 0.5516 | C × D × F | 0.73 | 0.49134 |
| Force × electrode | 4/36 | 0.7431 | 0.1857 | C × E × F | 3.61 | 0.01415 |
| Feedback × electrode | 2/18 | 0.7740 | 0.3870 | D × E × F | 3.99 | 0.03663 |
| Handedness × responding hand × force | 2/18 | 3.0563 | 1.5281 | B × C × F | 1.52 | 0.24405 |
| Handedness × responding hand × feeback | 1/9 | 0.0061 | 0.0061 | B × D × F | 0.01 | 0.94021 |
| Handedness × responding hand × electrode | 2/18 | 0.2532 | 0.1266 | B × E × F | 0.39 | 0.67788 |
| Handedness × force × feedback | 2/18 | 3.0563 | 1.5280 | C × D × F | 1.52 | 0.24405 |
| Handedness × force × electrode | 4/36 | 0.1405 | 0.0351 | C × E × F | 0.6835 | 0,60798 |
| Handedness × feedback × electrode | 2/18 | 0.4299 | 0.2149 | D × E × F | 2.21 | 0.13753 |
| Responding hand × force × feedback | 2/18 | 0.0346 | 0.0173 | B × C × D × F | 0.01 | 0.98860 |
| Responding hand × force × electrode | 4/36 | 1.3921 | 0.3480 | B × C × E × F | 10.52 | 0.00001 |
| Responding hand × feedback × electrode | 2/18 | 0.1104 | 0.0552 | B × D × E × F | 0.83 | 0.45122 |

| Source | df | | | Source | F | p |
|---|---|---|---|---|---|---|
| Force × feedback × electrode | 4/36 | 0.6279 | 0.1569 | C×D×E×F | 4.00 | 0.00872 |
| Handedness × responding hand × force × feedback | 2/18 | 1.2765 | 0.6382 | B×C×D×F | 0.42 | 0.66145 |
| Handedness × responding hand × force × electrode | 4/36 | 0.1753 | 0.0438 | B×C×E×F | 1.32 | 0.27891 |
| Handedness × responding hand × feedback × electrode | 2/18 | 0.6709 | 0.3354 | B×D×E×F | 5.05 | 0.01814 |
| Handedness × force × feedback × electrode | 4/36 | 0.2978 | 0.0744 | C×D×E×F | 1.89 | 0.13205 |
| Responding hand × force × feedback × electrode | 4/36 | 0.1480 | 0.0370 | B×C×D×E×F | 1.11 | 0.36654 |
| Handedness × responding hand × force × feedback × electrode | 4/36 | 0.1278 | 0.0319 | B×C×D×E×F | 0.95 | 0.44133 |
| Subjects (F) | | | | | | |

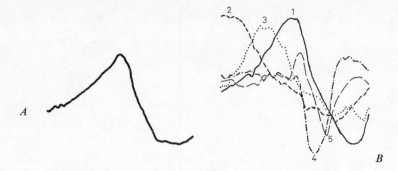

Fig. 7. *A* Grand average wave form obtained over all experimental conditions and all subjects (sum of 132 ERPs). *B* Factor loadings for each of the five factors extracted from a factor analysis of the ERP. The factors are labeled. Factor 1 is heavily loaded on variables associated with the overall wave form, factor 2 with the baseline, factor 3 with $N_1$, factor 4 with the $N_2$-$P_2$ transition points and factor 5 with component $P_2$.

The factor analysis is especially interesting in the light of the new information that it reveals concerning the late positive component ($P_2$) of the ERP. Table II presents an analysis of variance of factor scores on factor 5 ($P_2$) as the dependent variable. Both the presence and the absence of feedback have a significant effect on this factor. In fact, the factor scores for the two different feedback conditions are of equal amplitude but opposite polarity, positive and negative for the with and without feedback conditions, respectively. This provides a more direct assessment of the effect of feedback on the late positive component ($P_2$) which has too wide a range of latencies to be reduced to one characteristic measure. The responding hand × force × electrode interaction also has a significant effect ($p < 0.00001$) on the $P_2$ factor. Figure 8 shows a plot of these factor scores for $C_3$ and $C_4$ for right- and left-hand responses in each of the three force conditions. It is clear that the $P_2$ factor is asymmetric at higher force levels; the degree of asymmetry increasing as a function of increasing force. For right-handed responses, the post-response positivity ($P_2$) is consistently larger over the left sensorimotor condition while for left hand responses this holds true for all but the 0.25 force condition. This relation holds for both the with and without feedback conditions. We note that several of the third-order interactions are significant, but these will not be discussed in greater detail here.

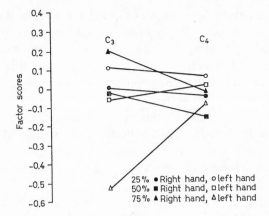

*Fig. 8.* Factor scores for the factor 5 or the $P_2$ component represented graphically for the $C_3$ and $C_4$ electrode positions for right- and left-hand responses, in each of the three force conditions.

## Discussion

*Handedness and contralateral dominance of $N_1$.* Movement-related potentials were recorded from eleven subjects squeezing a dynamometer, at three different force levels, with their right or left hand. The presence or absence of hemispheric asymmetry and the degree of such asymmetry appear to depend on the subject's handedness, the hand used for response and response force.

On the whole, the clearest degree of contralateral dominance appears in right-handed subjects, for whom the pre-motion cortical negativity ($N_1$ and part of $N_2$ as well) is significantly larger over the contralateral sensorimotor location. The asymmetry is reduced for left (non-dominant) hand responses. Left-handed subjects are not mirror image right handers. The left-handers studied here demonstrate contralateral dominance for right (non-dominant) hand responses and a greatly reduced sensorimotor asymmetry for left (dominant) hand responses. The large differences between right- and left-handed subjects is not without precedent in both the electrophysiological and behavioral literature. All investigators are in agreement that the left-handed population tends to be quite heterogeneous and can best be characterized as highly variable whatever the reported measure. Thus, while it is not surprising that the results of the left-handers in this study are different from those of the right-handers in that they show a reduced degree of hemispheric motor asymmetry preceding left-hand movements, an explanation for the right-hand contralateral dominance in left-handers is not readily apparent. We propose that a more extensive sampling of the left-handed population may provide several subgroups with different interhemispheric relations and a better estimate of the range of the left-handedness continuum.[1] Such data would also be more interpretable and informative when collected concurrently with several different measures (dichotic listening, inverted handwriting, horizontal scanning direction, orientation of drawn human profile, etc.) of the degree of cerebral dominance.

An especially interesting note concerning the data in both right- and left-handed subjects is that the absolute magnitude of the ipsilateral potential ($N_1$) is quite substantial. Uncrossed fiber systems of the brain allow a certain degree of bilateral sensory representation and motor control within each hemisphere. It has not only been shown that loss of ipsilateral function results in some sensorimotor deficits even when the contralateral hemisphere is intact, but also that although the majority of pyramidal cells fire with contralateral movement, some discharge only with ipsilateral movement [EVARTS, 1967]. It is difficult to disregard the size of the ipsilateral $N_1$ yet its amplitude is difficult to reconcile with the interpretation that the activity in the contralateral system may suppress or cancel the activity in the supposedly weaker ipsilateral system. A pattern of voluntary movements performed by one hand is often involuntarily altered when another movement has to be carried out simultaneously by the contralateral arm (or in fact any other part of the body) [COHEN, 1970]. Although there is an observed interaction between the limbs during bimanual voluntary activity, the cortical mechanism be it bilateral excitation or unilateral inhibition remains unknown for both the uni and bi-manual conditions.

*Force of response and $N_1$.* While response force does accentuate $N_1$ asymmetry, the absolute right-left asymmetry does not change with increasing force levels. Pilot data in our laboratory indicated that some minimal amount of force is necessary in order for the motor asymmetry to develop and be readily observable.

Our results are in accord with earlier reports (based on vertex data)

---

[1] Note added in proof: In the time since this paper was submitted, 25 additional sinistral subjects were tested. These new data essentially confirm this statement.

that increasing the force required to accomplish a response results in an increased CNV preceding the response [REBERT *et al.*, 1967; Low and McSherry, 1968]. As $N_1$ does not become more asymmetrical as a function of increased response force, our data are consistent with HILLYARD's [1973] two-component hypothesis which suggests that two sources contribute to the observed negativity: a lateralized slow negative wave specific to response-initiation and a relatively large, bilateral component, like the CNV, reflecting preparatory activity independent of the specific movement. Such a proposition is consistent with the notion that there is a family of task-related slow negative waves [DONCHIN *et al.*, 1972] of which the $N_1$ is but one member.

*Post-response components.* In this experiment, the force of response also has a significant effect on the $P_2$ component of the motor potential. Like $N_1$, $P_2$ is larger at the motor cortex contralateral to the activated limb, with the degree of asymmetry increasing as a function of increasing force. These findings are consistent with the suggestion that $P_2$ represents activity resulting from kinesthetic feedback (proprioceptive and somatosensory impulses) produced by the movement [BATES, 1951; VAUGHAN *et al.*, 1968; DEECKE *et al.*, 1969]. Part of the $P_2$ complexity reported by various investigators is probably a result of the confounding effect of a feedback associated with the completion of a movement or the achievement of a given output level. Our data indicate that with a more explicit feedback manipulation, there are substantial changes in the shape of $P_2$. The more peaked positivity seen in the feedback condition can be attributed either (1) to a possible superposition of various EP components onto the motor potential $P_2$ or (2) to the generation of a potential similar to the P300 resulting from the resolution of response parameter uncertainty provided by the feedback stimulus.

*Summary*

We report an experiment designed to assess the degree to which premovement negativity ($N_1$) is associated with the preparation to execute a response by determining the degree to which parameters of the response determine its waveform, amplitude, and distribution over the motor area. Eleven subjects were asked to perform self-paced, voluntary squeezes on a dynamometer at six to eight recording sessions. There were four independent variables: (1) the self-reported handedness of the subject (right or left); (2) the hand used in responding (right or left); (3) the amount of force required for any particular series of squeezes – each subject responded at three different force levels, preset at 25, 50, and 75% of his maximum determined separately for each hand, and (4) the presence or absence of an illuminated circle the extinguishing of which served to inform the subject when he has squeezed up to the required force level.

In right-handed subjects, $N_1$ was larger over the hemisphere contralateral to the responding hand. Left-handed subjects showed contralateral dominance when responding with the right hand and very little when responding with the left. Furthermore, while response force did accentuate $N_1$, the absolute right-left asymmetry did not change with increasing force levels.

These conclusions are supported by visual inspection, analysis of variance of $N_1$ area measures and a principal component analysis of the data. Our data are most consistent with a two-component hypothesis for the observed negativity: (1) a lateralized slow negative wave specific to response-initiation, and (2) a relatively large, bilateral component like the contingent negative variation, reflecting preparatory activity independent of the specific movement.

## Acknowledgments

This report is based in part on the data of a MA thesis submitted by M. KUTAS at the University of Illinois. We gratefully acknowledge the aid and comments received from M. COLES, E. WILLIAMS, E. HEFFLEY, and R. HERNING. The research was supported by the Advanced Research Projects Agency of the Department of Defense under Contract No. DAHC 15 73 C 0318, as well as by the University of Illinois Research Board and NIH Training Grant No. 5-TO1-MH-10715.

## References

BATES, J. A.: Electrical activity of the cortex accompanying movement. J. Physiol., Lond. *113:* 240–257 (1951).

COHEN, J.: Very slow brain potentials relating to expectancy in the CNV; in DONCHIN and LINDSLEY Average evoked potentials, methods, results and evaluations, NASA SP-191, pp. 143–198 (US Government Printing Office, Washington 1969).

COHEN, J. and WALTER, W. G.: The interaction of responses in the brain to semantic stimuli. Psychophysiology *2:* 187–196 (1966).

COHEN, L.: Interaction between limbs during bimanual voluntary activity. Brain *93:* 259–272 (1970).

DEECKE, L.; SCHEID, P., and KORNHUBER, H. H.: Distribution of readiness potential, pre-motion positivity and motor potential of the human cerebral cortex preceding voluntary finger movements. Expl Brain Res. *7:* 158–168 (1969).

DONCHIN, E.: A multivariate approach to the analysis of average evoked potentials. Trans. Bio-Med. Engng *13:* 131–139 (1966).

DONCHIN, E.; GERBRANDT, L. K.; LEIFER, L., and TUCKER, L.: Is the contingent negative variation contingent on a motor response. Psychophysiology *9:* 178–188 (1972).

DONCHIN, E.; KUBOVY, M.; KUTAS, M.; JOHNSON, R., and HERNING, R. I.: Graded changes in evoked response (P300) amplitude as a function of cognitive activity. Percept. Psychophys. *14:* 319–324 (1973).

DONCHIN, E. and LINDSLEY, D. B.: Average evoked potentials and reaction times to visual stimulus. Electroenceph. clin. Neurophysiol. *20:* 217–223 (1966).

EVARTS, E. V.: Relation of pyramidal tract activity to force exerted during a voluntary movement. J. Neurophysiol. *30:* 14–27 (1967).

GERBRANDT, L. K.; GOFF, W. R., and SMITH, D. B.: Distribution of the human average movement potential. Electroenceph. clin. Neurophysiol. *34:* 461–474 (1973).

GILDEN, L.; VAUGHAN, H. G., jr., and COSTA, L. D.: Summated human EEG potentials with voluntary movements. Electroenceph. clin. Neurophysiol. *20:* 433–438 (1966).

HILLYARD, S. A.: The CNV and human behavior. Electroenceph. clin. Neurophysiol. Suppl. *33:* 161–171 (1973).

IRWIN, D. A.; KNOTT, J. R.; McADAM, D. W., and REBERT, C. S.: Motivational determinants of 'the contingent negative variation'. Electroenceph. clin. Neurophysiol. *21:* 538–543 (1966).

JASPER, H. H.: Report of the committee on methods of clinical examination in electroencephalography. Electroenceph. clin. Neurophysiol. *10:* 370–375 (1958).

KORNHUBER, H. H. und DEECKE, L.: Hirnpotentialänderungen bei Willkürbewegungen und passiven Bewegungen des Menschen: Bereitschaftspotential und reafferente Potentiale. Pflügers Arch. ges. Physiol. *284:* 1–17 (1965).

KUTAS, M. and DONCHIN, E.: Studies of squeezing. The effects of handedness, the responding hand and response force on the contralateral dominance of the readiness potential. Science *186:* 545–548 (1974).

LOW, M. D.; BORDA, R. P.; FROST, J. D., jr., and KELLAWAY, P.: Surface-negative, slow-potential shift associated with conditioning in man. Neurology, Minneap. *16:* 771–782 (1966).

LOW, M. D. and McSHERRY, J. W.: Further observations of psychological factors involved in CNV genesis. Electroenceph. clin. Neurophysiol. *25:* 203–207 (1968).

McCALLUM, C.: The contingent negative variation as a cortical sign of attention in man; in EVANS and MULHOLLAND Attention in neurophysiology, pp. 40–63 (Butterworth, London 1969).

OLDFIELD, R. C.: The assessment and analysis of handedness. The Edinburgh inventory. Neuropsychologia *9:* 97–113 (1971).

OTTO, D. A. and LEIFER, L. J.: The effect of modifying response and performance feedback parameters on the CNV in human. Electroenceph. clin. Neurophysiol. Suppl. *33:* 29–37 (1973).

PETERS, J. F.; KNOTT, J. R., and MILLER, S. I.: Response variables and magnitude of the contingent negative variation. Electroenceph. clin. Neurophysiol. *29:* 608–611 (1970).

REBERT, C. S.; McADAM, D. W.; KNOTT, J. R., and IRWRIN, D. A.: Slow potential changes in human brain related to level of motivation. J. comp. physiol. Psychol. *63:* 20–23 (1967).

VAUGHAN, H. G., jr.: The relationship of brain activity to scalp recordings of event-related potentials; in DONCHIN and LINDSLEY Average evoked potentials, methods, results and evaluations, NASA SP-191, pp. 45–95 (US Government Printing Office, Washington 1969).

VAUGHAN, H. G., jr.; COSTA, L. D., and RITTER, W.: Topography of the human motor potential. Electroenceph. clin. Neurophysiol. *25:* 1–10 (1968).

WALTER, W. G.: Slow potential waves in the human brain associated with expectancy, attention and decision. Arch. Psychiat. NervKrankh. *206:* 309–322 (1964).

WALTER, W. G.; COOPER, R.; ALDRIDGE, V. J.; McCALLUM, W. C., and WINTER, A. L.: Contingent negative variation: an electric sign of sensori-motor association and expectancy in human brain. Nature, Lond. *203:* 380–384 (1964).

WEINBERG, H.: The contingent negative variation: its relation to feedback and expectant attention. Electroenceph. clin. Neurophysiol. Suppl. *33:* 219–228 (1973.)

Prof. EMANUEL DONCHIN, Department of Psychology, University of Illinois, *Champaign, IL 61820* (USA). Tel. (217) 333 3384.

Attention, Voluntary Contraction and Event-Related Cerebral Potentials.
Prog. clin. Neurophysiol., vol. 1, Ed. J. E. Desmedt, pp. 211–230 (Karger, Basel 1977)

# Slow Potential Components of
# Stimulus, Response and Preparatory Processes in Man

## A Multiple Linear Regression Model

D. A. Otto, V. A. Benignus, L. J. Ryan and L. J. Leifer

Environmental Protection Agency, University of North Carolina,
Chapel Hill, N.C.

Although negative slow potential (SP) shifts preceding motor and mental acts have been studied extensively, little effort has been made to elaborate SP changes during the motor act itself. We observed a large decrement in contingent negative variation (CNV) amplitude when a sustained motor response was superimposed on the S1-S2 interstimulus interval [Otto and Leifer, 1973a]. Results of a later study indicated that this decrement varied directly with the magnitude of response [Otto and Leifer, 1973b]. Results of the present study suggest that the observed CNV decrement was due to a prolonged positive shift arising during sustained motor response.

A three-stimulus paradigm was used to differentiate SP patterns associated with preparation for and execution of sustained motor response. Preparatory and holding intervals of varying length were employed to delineate waveforms associated with each component process. A control task was also included to examine SP changes during isometric motor response without external cues. Systematic manipulation of stimulus and response parameters permitted us to derive a simple additive model of negative preparatory and positive response-related components to account for the data. The model contains four predictor variables: (1) late positive component (LPC) of the visual evoked potential (VEP); (2) CNV; (3) readiness potential (RP), and (4) a positive response component (PRC).

## Methods

Ten right-handed male subjects aged 18–45 participated in the study. Geometric forms, presented on an IEE one-plane display device served as visual stimuli.

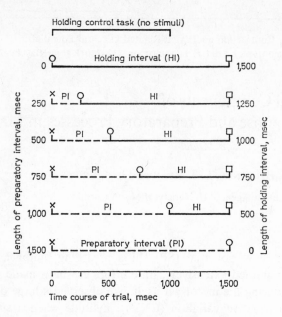

*Fig. 1.* Schema of experimental conditions. In the holding control task, subjects pressed and held 5 buttons down for 1 sec estimated without external cues. Visual stimuli were used in other conditions as cues to initiate a preparatory interval (×), to initiate a holding interval by pressing buttons (O), and to release buttons (□). Symbols correspond to actual geometric shapes used. Conditions are referred to by the length of the preparatory interval (i.e. in condition Ø there was no preparatory interval). In condition 1,500, subjects pressed and released buttons immediately following a single imperative stimulus (O).

Figure 1 illustrates the experimental design. Each subject completed 7 blocks of trials separated by 2-min rest intervals. Presentation of experimental conditions was counterbalanced to control for serial order effects. In the motor control task, subjects simultaneously pressed 5 finger buttons for an estimated 1-sec interval, counting slowly to 10 between trials. In the remaining conditions, trials consisted of 3 stimuli delineating preparatory (PI) and holding intervals (HI) varying in 250 msec increments such that PI + HI always equalled 1,500 msec. Random intertrial intervals 4–14 sec in length were used. In order to minimize eye movements, subjects fixated a cross in the center of the display.

EEG recordings were obtained with Beckman biopotential electrodes at Fz, Cz, and Pz referred to linked ears. Eye movements were recorded with diagonal bipolar placements above the inner canthus and below the outer canthus of the right eye. EEG and EOG were recorded on magnetic tape using an Ampex DAS-100 system with FM amplifiers set at a bandpass of 0.1–50 Hz. Analog data were digitized at 16 msec/point and averaged off-line with LINC-8 and PDP-12 computers. Eye movement artifact was minimized by: (1) requiring subjects to fixate; (2) inverting and subtracting EOG differentially from each EEG channel by means of dual input summing amplifiers[1], and (3) automatically rejecting trials containing large eye movements. Data were quantified by computing mean amplitudes, relative to a 1-sec pretrial baseline, of 8 successive 256-msec epochs.

## *Results*

*Non-cued holding task.* Slow potentials time-locked to key-press (KP) and key-release (KR) during the non-cued holding task are shown in figure 2. Summary averages were computed from 10 individual averages containing 20 trials each. Components preceding and accompanying the initiation of response are portrayed in KP averages. Since the task required subjects to estimate the duration of a 1-sec interval without external cues, considerable intra- and intersubject variability in the length of holding was observed. SPs accompanying the termination of response, therefore, are more accurately reflected in KR averages.

Three components of movement-related potentials described by VAUGHAN *et al.* [1968] and DEECKE *et al.* [1969] are evident in the vertex KP average. A slowly incrementing negative shift – the RP or $N_1$ component – commenced about 1 sec prior to movement. Pre-motion positivity ($P_1$) was not consistently observed in individual averages. An abrupt increase in the slope of $N_1$ (about 100 msec before movement at Cz) indicated the onset of the $N_2$ component. Note that a *positive* shift commenced at Pz contemporaneous with $N_2$ onset. A large positive shift ($P_2$), peaking 250–400 msec after KP onset, was observed at all recording sites. A prominent feature of this large positive shift, not emphasized in previous reports, was the prolongation of the waveform during sustained response. The waveform clearly persisted after the initiation of motor activity, although the shape and duration could not be specified precisely due to variability in the length of holding.

Averages triggered from the key-release mechanogram (fig. 2) suggest that the positive wave persisted throughout the holding interval at Fz and beyond KR at Pz. In fact, KR averages show that another positive

---

[1] Inputs to summing amplifiers had inverters and adjustable gains for selection of appropriate gain factors to balance out eye movement artifact at different scalp locations. EOG compensation factors were determined visually for each subject and recording site by simultaneously displaying EOG, raw EEG, and compensated EEG on an oscilloscope.

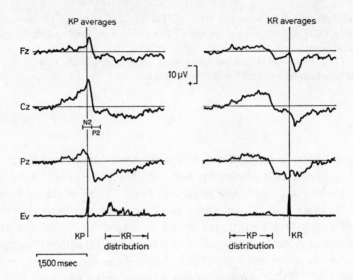

*Fig. 2.* Grand averages of SPs observed during the non-cued holding task in 10 subjects. KP and KR averages triggered from the onset of KP and KR mechanograms, respectively. Mean amplitudes of $N_2$ and $P_2$ components computed for 256-msec intervals as shown. Data digitized at 16 msec/point.

shift, maximal frontally, accompanied the termination of motor activity. Regrettably, EMG activity from responding muscles was not recorded. It is likely that EMG activity persisted briefly after KR, a factor which might account for the continuation of positivity at Pz.

In order to assess the topographical distribution of negative and positive response-related components, the mean amplitude of two consecutive 256-msec epochs, encompassing the $N_2$ and $P_2$ peaks, respectively, was measured with respect to baseline as shown in figure 2. $N_2$ was greater at Cz ($-15.5\ \mu$V) than Fz ($-6.7\ \mu$V) or Pz ($-2.6\ \mu$V) (Wilcoxon T = 5, N = 10, p = 0.02, and T = 0, N = 10, p<0.01, respectively).[2] $P_2$ was larger at Pz (13.5 $\mu$V) than Cz (3.8 $\mu$V; T = 4, N = 10, p<0.02) and Fz (4.4 $\mu$V) although the latter comparison failed to reach significance. $N_2$ thus had a more anterior distribution than $P_2$.

[2] Prior to making Wilcoxon comparisons, the null hypothesis of equal values at the 3 electrode sites was rejected on the basis of Friedman 2-way ANOVA ($\chi r^2$ = 9.8, N = 10, p<0.01).

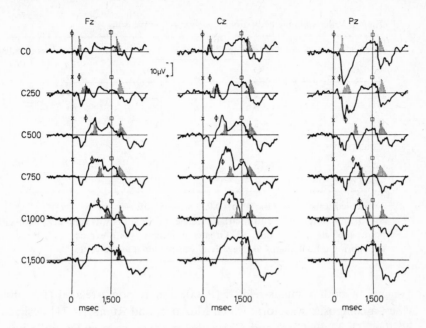

*Fig. 3.* Grand averages for cued-response conditions. Symbols as in figure 1. KP and KR histograms, plotted vertically along baseline, indicate distribution of response relative to stimulus events. Cnnn indicates length of preparatory interval in msec.

*Cued-response conditions.* The effect of superimposing a sustained motor response of varying length on a signaled 1,500-msec interval is illustrated in figure 3. Condition 1,500 (C1,500) corresponds to a standard CNV-eliciting situation with a brief KP required after a fixed 1,500-msec foreperiod. A characteristic rectangular negative wave was observed during C1,500. CØ constituted an opposite extreme with key-pressing required throughout the 1,500-msec interval. Table I shows the mean negative amplitude averaged across a $^3/_4$-sec interval preceding S2 in these conditions. The magnitude of negativity during CØ compared to C1,500 was significantly reduced at all recording sites. Table I also indicates that negative shifts were maximal at the vertex, a consistent finding in all cued-response conditions.

The pattern of SP shifts during S1-S2-S3 intervals of remaining conditions varied systematically in relation to stimulus-response contingencies. A large positive shift appeared in conjunction with the initiation of keypressing. This positive shift presumably contained late positive com-

*Table I.* Wilcoxon matched-pairs signed-ranks comparisons

| Electrode | Mean amplitude, $\mu V$ | | T values (n=10): C1,500>CØ |
|---|---|---|---|
| | CØ | C1,500 | |
| Fz | −4.3 | −11.6 | 6*** |
| Cz | −7.3 | −19.5 | 0* |
| Pz | −2.4 | −11.7 | 2* |
| T values (n=10) | | | |
| Cz>Fz | 13 | 1* | |
| Cz>Pz | 5** | 0* | |

Two-tailed tests: * $p<0.01$; ** $p=0.02$; *** $p=0.05$.
Mean amplitude, relative to pretrial baseline, of SP shifts was computed across 48 points (768 msec) preceding S2. Greater negativity was observed at all recording sites during C1,500 than CØ. Negativity was maximal at the vertex.

ponents of both stimulus-related (P300) and response-related (P₂) processes, a composite waveform which MCADAM and RUBIN [1971] designated the 'P302'. In C500 and C750, this positive wave at Fz and Cz appeared to be nested within a longer negative shift encompassing the entire 1,500-msec S1-S3 period.

The temporal relationship of SP changes and motor response is illustrated in figure 3. KP and KR histograms are plotted on the baseline of each average. Positive waves associated with key pressing commenced earliest at Pz. This relationship is shown more clearly in the following section in which a simple subtractive procedure is used to partial out the effect of sustained motor activity from the negative CNV-like shift presumed to span the 1,500-msec interstimulus interval in all cued-response conditions.

*Differential waveforms.* Since the stimulus-response contingencies of C1,500 correspond to a classical CNV-eliciting situation, C1,500 waveforms may be used as CNV standards for comparison with other conditions. The effect of superimposing a motor act of varying length may then be assessed by subtracting summary averages of CØ, C250, C500, C750, and C1,000 from the C1,500 standards. The resultant differential waveforms presumably represent the contribution of stimulus-response processes superimposed on the underlying CNV.

Differential waveforms plotted with polarity relative to C1,500 are shown in figure 4. These plots depict negative components preceding or

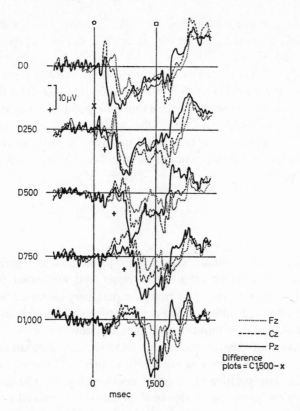

*Fig. 4.* Differential plots obtained by subtracting summary averages of CØ, C250, ..., C1,000 from C1,500 waveforms. Differential waveforms (Dnnn) reflect the residual contribution to observed SPs of stimulus-response events superimposed on a classic CNV-eliciting situation represented by C1,500. Polarity is relative to C1,500 waveforms.

accompanying the onset of response and positive shifts persisting during response. Negative components were largest at the vertex. The negative differential wave in D0 and D250 was similar in shape, time course, and topography to the $N_2$ component observed during non-cued response. Differential pre-response negativity in D500, D750, and D1,000 incremented more gradually similar to the $N_1$ component observed in the non-cued response condition. Differential positivity commenced earliest, reached maximal amplitude, and decayed earliest at Pz. The duration of this waveform was directly proportional to the length of the holding interval. Differential positivity presumably corresponds to the prolonged $P_2$ wave observed in the non-cued response condition. Both the negative and positive components of D750, in particular, closely resembled the KP averages obtained during non-cued response.

D250, D500, D750, and D1,000 waveforms contain positivity related to the imperative stimulus (S2) as well as the motor response. The KP imperative in CØ, however, occurred at the same time point as the warning stimulus in C1,500. Stimulus artifact in D0 waveforms, therefore, was minimal. Since the configuration of differential positivity in D0 was very similar to other conditions, the contribution of stimulus-related processes appeared to be negligible.

## Discussion

*Response-related slow potentials.* BATES [1951] described a negative shift commencing about 20 msec after EMG onset and attributed the wave to the 'arrival of afferent impulses from the periphery'. KORNHUBER and DEECKE [1965] observed both positive and negative shifts following a variety of hand, wrist, and foot movements. Since the slow potential patterns following active and passive movement were similar, KORNHUBER and DEECKE [1965] dismissed them as reafferent in origin. GILDEN *et al.* [1966] attributed the late positive component commencing 50–150 msec after EMG onset which 'persisted or slowly decayed with sustained contraction' to somatosensory or proprioceptive feedback from responding muscles. VAUGHAN *et al.* [1968] later designated this late positive wave as the $P_2$ component of the motor potential. The slow positive shift observed in the present motor task appears to be a prolongation of the $P_2$ wave. VAUGHAN *et al.* [1968] reported that $P_2$ was maximal over Rolandic cortex and decreased in amplitude postcentrally. VAUGHAN's 'P' measurement was made between $N_2$ and $P_2$ peaks, however, and probably reflected the distribution of $N_2$ rather than $P_2$. GERBRANDT *et al.* [1973] found a more posterior distribution of $P_2$ when amplitude was measured relative to a pre-$N_2$ baseline. We also found that the late positive shift during response was maximal postcentrally. The observed posterior gradient of response-related positivity is consistent with previous speculations that it reflects proprioceptive or kinesthetic input from responding musculature. Such information could be utilized by the cortex in maintaining tension in peripheral muscle spindles for the appropriate duration of response. The evidence, however, is inconclusive. The sustained positive shift may indeed not reflect peripheral input at all. VAUGHAN *et al.* [1970], for instance, found no change in motor-related potentials of monkeys following upper limb deafferentation. They speculated that kinesthetic feedback to the motor cortex may be blocked during motor discharge. Study of the somatosensory evoked potential also suggests that afferent input may be inhibited by movement. COQUERY *et al.* [1972] and HAZEMANN and LILLE [1976] observed a decrease in amplitude of the SEP during motor response. On the other hand, LEE and WHITE [1974] reported an increase in amplitude of the $N_3$ component of the SEP during active movement. The effect of movement on SEP is thus equivocal.

Proprioceptive feedback is thought to have an important role in the timing of motor response [cf. SCHMIDT, 1971]. The sustained positive shift could reflect a central timing mechanism rather than reafference, since time estimation was an integral part of the non-cued response task. MCADAM [1966] reported a slow *negative* shift at the vertex during time estimation but he did not record postcentrally. REBERT [1976] observed a prolonged positive shift in the parietal region during weight-pulling when induced muscle tension was minimal (0–15 lb.). When tension was increased, however, the parietal region shifted negative. Since external stimuli were used to signal the onset and termination of pulling, the paradigm may have served as an extended CNV-eliciting situation. The motoric relationship of slow potentials observed by REBERT is uncertain since non-cued control conditions were not run.

Preliminary investigation [OTTO and BENIGNUS, 1975] of slow positive shifts during isometric contraction indicates that these waveforms are not proportional to the length or force of contraction and are bilaterally symmetrical. Nor can sustained positive shifts be attributed to central timing processes: slow negative shifts were observed during time estimation without isometric contraction, consistent with MCADAM [1966]. These results do not support the reafferent or central timing hypotheses. Further study is needed to determine the functional significance of slow positive shifts observed on the scalp during motor response.

*Interaction of component processes.* OTTO and LEIFER [1973a] found that the magnitude of CNV was substantially reduced during sustained motor response signaled at fixed intervals. A randomized intertrial interval was used in the present study to control for pretrial anticipatory effects. A large decrement in CNV was again observed during sustained response. CNV reduction, in this case, cannot be dismissed as a pretrial anticipatory artifact.

Reduction in the amplitude of CNV during response could be an indirect result of the distracting nature of the imposed motor act. MCCALLUM and WALTER [1968] and TECCE and SCHEFF [1969] have shown that CNV magnitude decreases when distracting events are present during the CNV interval. Results of the motor task suggest an alternative explanation. When subjects were required to press and hold for 1 sec without external cues, a prolonged positive shift was observed during response. When holding was superimposed on a cued 1,500-msec interval, a similar positive shift was observed during the response segment. A simple subtractive procedure was used to isolate the contribution of sustained motor activity to observed waveforms in cued response conditions. Differential waveforms obtained in this manner closely resembled SP patterns observed during the non-cued motor task. The similarity of D750 waveforms was particularly striking. Results of the motor task and subtractive procedure indicate, therefore, that the decrement in CNV magnitude previously reported [OTTO and LEIFER, 1973a, b] was due to the interaction of negative preparatory and positive response-related potentials rather than distraction. The precise relationship of positive shifts to motor activity, however, remains obscure.

MCCALLUM and PAPAKOSTOPOULOS [1972] also found a decrement in CNV amplitude when a sustained motor response was initiated during an S1-S2 interval. When the CNV interval was imposed on a background of sustained response, however, no decrement was observed. They concluded that the decrement was due to the initiation of motor activity rather than the maintenance of response *per se*. This conclusion is questionable in light of the persistence of postcentral positivity during the non-cued response task in the present study. Response-related positivity appears to reflect more than the simple initiation of movement.

BORDA [1970], JARVILEHTO and FRUSTORFER [1970], and McSHERRY *et al.* [this volume] have suggested that the vertex CNV reflects multiple underlying neural processes which summate on the scalp. ROHRBAUGH *et al.* [1976], using a long interstimulus interval (4 sec), have distinguished two negative components – an early frontal stimulus-dependent wave and a later motor-preparatory Rolandic wave [SYNDULKO and LINDSLEY, this volume]. Results of the present study are fully consistent with the multiprocess view. It is necessary, therefore, to isolate and identify component processes in order to understand the functional significance of complex scalp-recorded SPs. A technique to differentiate component processes which overlap in time is described below.

## Theoretical Model

The complex SP waveforms observed in this study appear to be composite patterns containing several components. Four major components can be distinguished: (1) a late positive component (LPC) associated with the visual stimuli; (2) a slow incrementing negative shift preceding motor response corresponding to the RP; (3) a slow positive component occurring during motor response which we will designate the PRC, and (4) the CNV.

In order to obtain estimates of these components which would yield the best approximation of observed SP patterns, simplified templates of each component were constructed and fitted to the empirical data. Mathematically, the model can be expressed as:

$$\widehat{(CSP)}_t = \beta_1(CNV)_t + \beta_2(PRC)_t + \beta_3(RP)_t + \beta_4(LPC)_t \tag{1}$$

where $\widehat{(CSP)}_t$ is the estimated or predicted voltage of the complex SP at time t and the terms $(CNV)_t$, $(PRC)_t$, $(RP)_t$, and $(LPC)_t$ represent the estimated values of each component process at the same point in time. The terms $\beta_1$-$\beta_4$ are empirical weights fitted to the model by least squares methods.

*Estimates of the four components.* In order to fit equation 1 to the observed value of $(CSP)_t$, it was necessary to obtain unbiased estimates of each component. Estimates of (CNV), (PRC), and (RP) were derived from the present experiment. Since no adequate stimulus control condition was run, the LPC template was conceived simply as a positive triangular waveform peaking 300 msec after stimulus onset. A schematic representation of these components for each experimental condition is shown in figure 5.

The stimulus-response contingencies of condition 1,500 are equivalent to a standard CNV paradigm. The slow negative shift observed at the vertex during this condition (fig. 3) was therefore used as the CNV template. To simplify the template, the summary average was reduced to eight data points by computing the average amplitude of successive 256-msec segments commencing at S1 onset. These values are represented in figure 5 as bar-graph elements superimposed on the CNV template. RP and PRC templates were derived analogously from SP patterns observed during the non-cued motor control task (KP averages) at Cz and Pz, respectively.

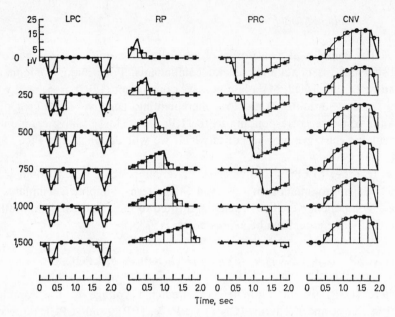

*Fig. 5.* Templates used to compute multiple regression of theoretical components to observed data. Components include: (1) late positive component (LPC) associated with each visual stimulus; (2) readiness potential (RP) preceding key press; (3) positive response component (PRC) accompanying pressing, and (4) contingent negative variation (CNV). Mean amplitudes of successive 1/4-sec epochs were calculated for each template as indicated by bar-graph elements. These values were used in regression analysis.

*Temporal position of components.* Component templates were positioned along the time axis in accordance with the temporal pattern of stimuli and motor responses in the six experimental conditions. Each row in figure 5 corresponds to one of the experimental conditions (0, 250, ..., 1,500). LPC components were assumed to peak 300 msec after each stimulus. Identical CNV components were hypothesized for all conditions commencing approximately 400 msec after S1 onset, continuing throughout the remainder of the 1,500-msec interstimulus interval, and decaying abruptly after the final stimulus.

Additional assumptions were required to construct RP components since the readiness potential by definition is elicited in the absence of stimuli. When stimuli were used to delimit an interval preparatory to response, we assumed that a neural process analogous to the RP commenced at the onset of the initial warning stimulus. Kornhuber and

DEECKE [1965], VAUGHAN *et al.* [1968] and others reported that the RP begins 1–2 sec before movement onset [DEECKE and KORNHUBER, this volume]. When response is signaled by an external cue, however, the RP duration may be considerably shorter. For instance, reaction time to auditory stimuli is usually on the order of 160–180 msec. For the purpose of the model, we assumed that the RP component commenced at S1 onset, regardless of the length of the preparatory interval. We further assumed that the RP component reached peak amplitude 350 msec after the onset of the imperative stimulus (S1 in CØ and S2 in C250–C1,500). This value was selected because reaction times averaged 350 msec across conditions. Finally, we assumed that the peak amplitude of the RP component was constant across experimental conditions. The slope of the RP component thus varied inversely with the length of the preparatory interval. The preparatory interval of C750 corresponded closely to the duration of the RP observed in the motor control task (fig. 2). The RP template for C750 was therefore constructed directly from the vertex summary KP average of the motor control task. RP components for other conditions were extrapolated from this template.

The RP template admittedly represents an extreme simplification of 'true' waveforms [cf. DEECKE and KORNHUBER, this volume]. It should be noted, however, that reduction of waveforms to 8 data points (representing consecutive 0.25-sec epochs) effectively filters out the fine detail of fast components.

The PRC template was also derived from the motor control task (parietal summary KP average), again assuming the peak amplitude of the PRC component to be constant across conditions. Since the PRC persisted beyond KR, the slope was assumed to be constant across conditions. The ascending limb of the PRC component was plotted as a continuation of the RP denouement.

*Fitting the model.* A multiple linear regression program (BMD 03R) [DIXON, 1970] was used to compute the set of weights $(\beta_1$-$\beta_4)$ which would yield the best approximation of observed complex slow potentials (CSPs). CSP values from summary averages were used as the criterion to which predictor waveforms were fitted. Criterion waveforms were represented by eight data points for each experimental condition as previously described. Analogous data sets depicted in figure 5 were entered for each of the 4 predictor variables. Predictor variables could now be regressed against observed criterion values to determine best fit weights for each experimental condition. We are more interested in a general solution across

*Table II.* Results of multiple regression analysis to determine best fit of theoretical components to observed data

| | Regression coefficients | | | | Multiple correlation | F value* |
|---|---|---|---|---|---|---|
| | LPC | RP | PRC | CNV | | |
| **a) 4-component model (vertex CNV template)** | | | | | | |
| Fz | 0.51 | 0.36 | 0.34 | 0.56 | 0.823 | 23.04 |
| Cz | 0.80 | 1.01 | 0.41 | 0.80 | 0.928 | 66.88 |
| Pz | 1.26 | −0.14 | 0.99 | 0.84 | 0.925 | 63.77 |
| **b) 4-component model (frontal CNV template)** | | | | | | |
| Fz | 0.29 | 0.01 | 0.42 | 1.07 | 0.898 | 44.83 |
| Cz | 0.57 | 0.73 | 0.35 | 1.22 | 0.914 | 54.32 |
| Pz | 1.14 | −0.09 | 0.65 | 0.80 | 0.811 | 20.63 |
| **c) 3-component model omitting RP (vertex CNV template)** | | | | | | |
| Fz | 0.57 | – | 0.53 | 0.61 | 0.812 | 28.37 |
| Cz | 0.97 | – | 0.96 | 0.93 | 0.884 | 52.24 |
| Pz | 1.24 | – | 0.91 | 0.82 | 0.854 | 85.96 |

* d.f. $= 4$; $6 < n < 43$ for *a* and *b*. d.f. $= 3$; $6 < n < 44$ for *c*. $p < 0.01$ for all F values.

conditions, however, than a unique solution for each individual condition. We want to compute a single set of weights (regression coefficients) which will define the best fit to all observed data. In other words, we wish to constrain the amplitude of predictor variables across conditions in order to obtain the most general solution of the model. A simple method used to achieve this goal was to join the waveforms for each of the 7 experimental conditions end-to-end to form a single continuous data string containing $6 \times 8 = 48$ values. This procedure was repeated for each electrode and each predictor variable.

Results of the multiple linear regression computation are presented in table II. Predicted CSPs were then constructed using equation 1. Plots of observed and predicted waveforms are shown in figure 6.

The accuracy of the model may be judged from the multiple correlations shown in table IIa. Squared correlation coefficients represent the amount of variance in the observed data accounted for by the predictor variables: 68.2, 86.1 and 85.6% for Fz, Cz, and Pz, respectively. These results suggest remarkably accurate prediction.

Since adjacent points in any observed or predicted waveform are correlated to an unknown degree, we cannot assume that the 48 data points

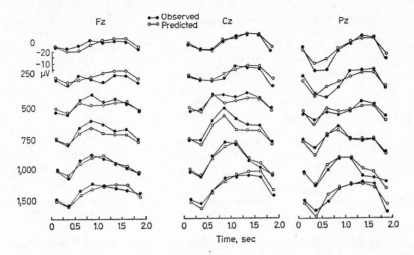

*Fig. 6.* Comparison of predicted and observed waveforms at frontal, central, and parietal recording sites. Template values were multiplied by regression coefficients and summed across components to obtain predicted waveforms. Component templates were assumed to be identical in shape, but differentially weighted in amplitude at the three scalp positions.

in each variable are independent. For this reason, no precise estimate of degrees of freedom (d.f.) is available for the model. We can estimate, however, that the denominator of the F-ratio has $6 < n < 43$ degrees of freedom with d.f. $= 4$ for the numerator [cf. GEISSER and GREENHOUSE, 1958]. Based on the most conservative estimate, the lowest observed correlation (Fz, r = 23.04, d.f. = 4.6) is significant at $p < 0.01$. The highest correlation was obtained at the vertex (r = 0.928, F = 66.88).

Partial correlations provide a more detailed picture of the variance accounted for by individual components of the model. The proportion of the total variance accounted for by each predictor variable, assuming that other variables are held constant, can be estimated from the squared partial correlation coefficients [GUILFORD, 1967, pp. 405–406]. Table IIIa shows, for instance, that the RP variable accounts for less than 10% of the variance in CSPs at Fz and less than 1% at Pz! The RP component contributed primarily to waveforms observed at the vertex, while the PRC contributed primarily to parietal waveforms. The CNV and LPC components, on the other hand, accounted for major portions of the variance at all three recording sites.

*Table III.* Partial correlation coefficients

|  | LPC | RP | PRC | CNV |
|---|---|---|---|---|
| a) 4-component model (vertex CNV template) | | | | |
| Fz | 0.532 | 0.258 | 0.324 | 0.693 |
| Cz | 0.713 | 0.607 | 0.391 | 0.815 |
| Pz | 0.844 | −0.102 | 0.715 | 0.824 |
| b) 4-component model (frontal CNV template) | | | | |
| Fz | 0.402 | 0.010 | 0.483 | 0.827 |
| Cz | 0.535 | 0.427 | 0.318 | 0.774 |
| Pz | 0.664 | −0.043 | 0.405 | 0.488 |

*Extension of the model.* Templates for CNV and RP were derived from vertex observations. The PRC template was based on the summary KP average at Pz. These circumstances contribute, no doubt, to the high correlations at Cz and Pz. Regression coefficients of theoretical components correspond well to the observed topographical distribution of the LPC, RP, and PRC. Weights of the CNV component, however, do not correspond directly with observed topography. The largest CNVs were consistently observed at the vertex, whereas the model yielded a slightly higher regression coefficient at Pz (0.84) than Cz (0.80). This discrepancy may be explained by the composite nature of the empirical waveform.

According to the model, the CSP preceding response contains both CNV and RP components. The model predicts, moreover, that RP contributes substantially to vertex CSPs, but very little to postcentral CSPs. Negativity observed at Pz may thus represent almost 'pure' CNV, while negativity observed at the vertex probably contains a large proportion of RP. The finding of peak negativity at the vertex in a classical CNV-eliciting situation requiring motor response may thus reflect the distribution of motor-related components ($N_1$ or $N_2$) rather than the CNV.

This conclusion is supported by evidence that the scalp distribution of CNV varies widely relative to task demands. COHEN [1969], MARSH *et al.* [1973] and RITTER *et al.* [this series] have reported a posterior shift in CNV distribution in tasks requiring cognitive processing or sensory discrimination in contrast to standard foreperiod or disjunctive reaction-time tasks. LEIFER *et al.* [1973] found that CNV was maximal at Pz during a complex probability learning task in which trials were initiated rather than terminated by button pressing. The consistent finding of maximal

CNV at the vertex in reaction-time studies may thus be an artifact of the RP component which contributes heavily to SPs recorded at this site.

Simplicity of the model permits facile modification of basic parameters and immediate determination of the consequences of the goodness of fit. For instance, if the shape of an observed waveform varies perceptibly across the scalp, one could construct multiple templates for that waveform. Critical features, such as peak latency or slope could be varied in accordance with observed differences.

The difference in shape of the CNV at frontal and central recording sites provides an interesting example. The CNV tended to rise more abruptly and peak earlier at Fz than Cz. How well would the model fit if we constructed the CNV template from data observed at Fz rather than Cz? Table IIb illustrates the results. Regression coefficients maintained the same relative proportion across the scalp with the exception of the CNV component. Maximal weighting of this component shifted from Pz to Cz. Thus, the frontal CNV template provided a better approximation than the vertex template of the observed topography of component waveforms. On the other hand, the total amount of variance accounted for in the model was greater when the vertex CNV template was used. The decrease in predictive power of the model is illustrated for individual components in table IIIb. Each of the predictor variables accounted for less of the total variance when the frontal CNV template was substituted for the vertex template.

Can we draw any further implications from the model regarding the composite nature of observed waveforms? It has often been speculated that the CNV and RP reflect the same underlying neural process [WALTER, 1967]. This hypothesis may be evaluated by dropping one of these components. Multiple correlations dropped at all three recording sites with multiple correlation. Table IIc illustrates the result of omitting the RP component. Multiple correlations dropped at all three recording sites with the largest decrease occurring at Pz. Furthermore, the regression coefficients of the PRC component no longer conformed to observed topography.

Predictive power of the model, therefore, was substantially improved by employing both the RP and PRC components. This finding suggests that the CNV and RP contribute differentially to SP patterns recorded over different parts of the brain and probably reflect different generator mechanisms. The results further suggest that the CNV and RP are confounded at the vertex when a motor response is required at the end of an expectancy interval.

The proportion of variance in observed data accounted for by the multiple regression model is impressive. The results, in general, provided strong evidence of the composite nature of event-related SPs recorded from the scalp. The simple additive nature of the model is quite compatible with the spatial-averaging, volume conduction characteristics of the cranium. It should be noted that the data were greatly simplified by averaging across successive 256-msec epochs, a crude smoothing process which helped reduce variance. The model is by no means restricted to such simple waveforms. Extension of the model to more complex samples will provide a better index of its utility in the study of SPs. In summary, the model appears to provide a promising method for differentiating the functional components of complex event-related potentials of the brain.

## Summary

This study was undertaken to elaborate slow potential patterns associated with the preparation for and execution of sustained motor response. Preparatory and holding intervals of varying length were used to examine the interaction of the contingent negative variation (CNV), the readiness potential (RP), and the late positive component (LPC) of the sensory evoked response. The topographical distribution of motor-related potentials at frontal, central, and parietal midline sites was also assessed in cued and non-cued response conditions.

A slow positive response-related component (PRC) was observed during sustained button-pressing in the absence of external stimuli. When sustained motor response was superimposed on a CNV-eliciting interval, a decrement in negativity was observed. The CNV, RP, LPC, and PRC appear to summate linearly in complex slow potentials recorded on the scalp.

A multiple regression model was constructed to evaluate the contribution of CNV, RP, LPC, and PRC components to observed waveforms. The model provided a remarkably accurate approximation of empirical waveforms and accounted for 68–86% of the variance in observed data. Results suggest that the CNV and RP contribute differentially to slow potentials over different parts of the brain and probably reflect separate generator mechanisms. The model thus offers a promising method for teasing apart the functional components of complex event-related potentials of the brain.

## Acknowledgments

The authors are indebted to R. M. PATTON, E. HUFF, and J. H. KNELSON for support and to D. NAGLE for advice on the regression model. This study was conducted at NASA-Ames Research Center where the senior author held an NRC Research Associateship.

*References*

BATES, J. A. V.: Electrical activity of the cortex accompanying movement. J. Physiol., Lond. *113:* 240–257 (1951).

BORDA, R. P.: The effect of altered drive states on the contingent negative variation in rhesus monkeys. Electroenceph. clin. Neurophysiol. *29:* 173–180 (1970).

COHEN, J.: Very slow brain potentials relating to expectancy: the CNV; in DONCHIN and LINDSLEY Average evoked potentials: methods, results and evaluations, NASA SP-191, pp. 143–198 (US Government Printing Office, 1969).

COHEN, J. and WALTER, W. G.: The interaction of responses in the brain to semantic stimuli. Psychophysiology *2:* 187–196 (1966).

COQUERY, J. C.; COULMANCE, M. et LERON, M. L.: Modifications des potentials évoqués corticaux somesthétiques durant des mouvements et passifs chez l'homme. Electroenceph. clin. Neurophysiol. *33:* 269–276 (1972).

DEECKE, L.; SCHEID, P., and KORNHUBER, H. H.: Distributions of readiness potential, pre-motion positivity, and motor potential of human cerebral cortex preceding voluntary finger movements. Expl Brain Res. *7:* 158–168 (1969).

DIXON, W. J. (ed.): BMD Biomedical Computer Programs (University of California Press, Los Angeles 1970).

GEISSER, S. and GREENHOUSE, S. W.: An extension of Box's results on the use of the F distribution in multivariate analysis. Am. Math. Stat. *29:* 885–891 (1958).

GERBRANDT, L. K.; GOFF, W. R., and SMITH, D. B.: Distribution of the human average movement potential. Electroenceph. clin. Neurophysiol. *34:* 461–474 (1973).

GILDEN, L.; VAUGHAN, H. G., and COSTA, L. D.: Summated human EEG potentials with voluntary movement. Electroenceph. clin. Neurophysiol. *20:* 433–438 (1966).

GUILFORD, J. P.: Fundamental statistics in psychology and education; 4th ed. (McGraw-Hill, New York 1965).

HAZEMANN, P. and LILLE, F.: Somatosensory evoked potentials, attention and voluntary self-paced movements; in McCALLUM and KNOTT The responsive brain, pp. 111–113 (Wright, Bristol 1976).

JARVILEHTO, R. and FRUHSTORFER, H.: Differentiation between slow cortical potential associated with motor and mental acts in man. Expl Brain Res. *4:* 309–317 (1970).

KORNHUBER, H. H. und DEECKE, L.: Hirnpotentialänderungen bei Willkürbewegungen und passiven Bewegungen des Menschen: Bereitschaftspotential und reafferente Potentiale. Pflügers Arch. ges. Physiol. *284:* 1–17 (1965).

LEE, R. C. and WHITE, D. G.: Modification of the human somatosensory evoked response during voluntary movement. Electroenceph. clin. Neurophysiol. *36:* 53–62 (1974).

LEIFER, L. J.; OTTO, D. A.; HART, S. G., and HUFF, E. M.: Slow potential correlates of predictive behavior during a complex learning task; in McCALLUM and KNOTT The responsive brain, pp. 65–70 (Wright, Bristol 1976).

MARSH, G. R.; POON, L. W., and THOMPSON, L. W.: Some relationships between CNV, P300, and task demands; in McCALLUM and KNOTT The responsive brain, pp. 122–125 (Wright, Bristol 1976).

MCADAM, D. W.: Slow potential changes recorded from human brain during learning of a temporal interval. Psychon. Sci. *6:* 435–436 (1966).

MCADAM, D. W. and RUBIN, E. H.: Readiness potential, vertex positive wave, contingent negative variation and accuracy of perception. Electroenceph. clin. Neurophysiol. *30:* 511–517 (1971).

MCCALLUM, W. C. and WALTER, W. G.: The effects of attention and distraction on the contingent negative variation in normal and neurotic subjects. Electroenceph. clin. Neurophysiol. *25:* 319–329 (1968).

OTTO, D. A. and BENIGNUS, V. A.: Slow positive shifts during sustained motor activity in humans. Electroenceph. clin. Neurophysiol. *38:* 542P (1975).

OTTO, D. A. and LEIFER, L. J.: The effect of modifying response and performance feedback parameters on the CNV in humans. Electroenceph. clin. Neurophysiol. Suppl. *33:* 29–37 (1973a).

OTTO, D. A. and LEIFER, L. J.: Effects of varying the magnitude, duration and speed of motor response on the contingent negative variation. Electroenceph. clin. Neurophysiol. *34:* 695P (1973b).

REBERT, C.; BERRY, R., and MERLO, J.: DC potential consequences of induced muscle tension. Effects on contingent negative variation; in MCCALLUM and KNOTT The responsive brain, pp. 130–131 (Wright, Bristol 1976).

ROHRBAUGH, J. W.; SYNDULKO, K., and LINDSLEY, D. B.: Brain wave components of the contingent negative variation in humans. Science *191:* 1055–1057 (1976).

SCHMIDT, R. A.: Proprioception and the timing of motor responses. Psychol. Bull. *76:* 383–393 (1971).

TECCE, J. J. and SCHEFF, N. M.: Attention reduction and suppressed direct-current potentials in the human brain. Science *164:* 331–333 (1969).

VAUGHAN, H. G.; COSTA, L. D., and RITTER, R.: Topography of the human motor potential. Electroenceph. clin. Neurophysiol. *25:* 1–10 (1968).

VAUGHAN, H. G.; GROSS, E. G., and BOSSOM, J.: Cortical motor potential in monkeys before and after upper limb deafferentiation. Expl Neurol. *26:* 253–262 (1970).

WALTER, W. G.: Slow potential changes in the human brain associated with expectancy, decision and intention. Electroenceph. clin. Neurophysiol. Suppl. *26:* 123–130 (1967).

Dr. DAVID A. OTTO, Environmental Protection Agency, University of North Carolina, Mason Farm Road, *Chapel Hill, NC 27514* (USA). Tel. (919) 966 2321.

Attention, Voluntary Contraction and Event-Related Cerebral Potentials.
Prog. clin. Neurophysiol., vol. 1, Ed. J. E. DESMEDT, pp. 231–241 (Karger, Basel 1977)

# Analysis of Event-Related Slow Potentials in Primates[1]

JOSEPH W. McSHERRY, ROBERT P. BORDA and JOHN J. HABLITZ

Department of Neurophysiology, Methodist Hospital, and Department of
Physiology, Baylor College of Medicine, Houston, Tex.

Several years ago, data from this and other laboratories suggested a
theoretical basis for the generation and evolution of event-related slow
potentials (SPs). This explanation suggested that: (1) the contingent negative variation (CNV) is, in fact, a composite of several discrete SPs; (2) it
consists of both somatic hyperpolarization (extracellular-positive shifts)
and dendritic depolarization (superficial negativity); (3) the former presumably is mediated by cortico-cortical connections and the latter by non-
specific arousal afferents, and (4) as learning progresses, the CNV under-
goes an evolution from representing a widespread priming of frontal cortex to a priming which is more circumscribed, involving primarily the pre-
motor region. Data presented in this book and elsewhere suggests further
refinement of this hypothetical model.

The conclusion that the CNV recorded from the scalp must represent
spatial summation from multiple sources of SPs comes from cortical recordings in both man [WALTER, 1968] and monkey [McSHERRY and BOR-
DA, 1973], where it had been observed that isolated 'islands' of SP activity were found interspersed among relatively inactive areas.

The neuronal mechanisms underlying the elaboration of the CNV
were postulated [McSHERRY, 1973] on the basis of observations of the intracortical distribution of negative and positive SPs [McSHERRY, unpublished doctoral dissertation; McSHERRY and BORDA, 1973] and an extrap-
olation of previously described relationships between EEG phenomena

[1] Supported in part by Grants NGR 44-003-001 from the National Aeronau-
tics and Space Administration and HL 05435 from the National Heart and Lung Institute, NIH, USPHS.

and intracellular events [CREUTZFELDT *et al.*, 1966]. It was hypothesized that a deep positive shift was induced by cortico-cortical connections with resultant axosomatic inhibition and possibly a supplemental decrease in excitatory input from the specific thalamocortical afferents, with a subsequent positive shift in the depth. The superficial negativity was presumed to have been induced by nonspecific excitatory projections. Data giving evidence for these pathways comes from numerous authors and is summarized in a previous paper [McSHERRY, 1973]. In the light of the observations of YINGLING and SKINNER [this volume] on gating in the thalamic nucleus reticularis (NR), one may hypothesize a pathway through which the decrease in specific thalamocortical activity is mediated. Fibers originating in pre-motor cortex project to NR by way of the inferior thalamic preduncle (ITP). Activation of these fibers could act to excite specific regions of NR, regions which are predominantly inhibitory in action, and result in a net decrease in outflow to the cortex from the specific sensory nuclei of the thalamus. This inhibition of specific thalamic input to cortical cells would produce a net decrease in somatic depolarization and a subsequent depth-positive SP shift. That cerebrocortical cells do alter their firing rate during the S1-S2 interval has been shown previously [FROST and LOW, 1967].

The evolution of the CNV from being a phenomenon involving widespread areas of the frontal lobe to one which is limited more to the pre-motor cortex has been observed in the rhesus monkey model in several independent investigations [BORDA, 1970; REBERT, 1972; HABLITZ, 1973; McSHERRY, unpublished doctoral dissertation]. The significance of this evolution is hypothesized to be that, as learning takes place, the organism first observes that there is a significant probability that S2 will be preceded by another stimulus (S1), a stimulus which the organism has not yet defined. While affirming this relationship between S1 and S2 and delineating the character of S1, wide areas of cortex are primed for the anticipated response. Later, when the direct relationship between S1 and S2 is established, only those areas of cortex needed for specific reception of these stimuli and discrete execution of the response need to be primed, and these areas appear to be located in pre-motor cortex in the rhesus monkey. In particular, Brodmann's area 6, in which certain integrated movements appear to be organized, and the area of sulcus principalis, which has been shown to be critical to storage and retrieval of information in a delayed-response task [STAMM and ROSEN, 1969], show well-developed CNVs late in learning. Area 4, or motor cortex, shows little activity in overtrained monkeys in the S1-S2 interval, but shows a marked surface-positive potential prior to the response (and reward).

Because the data supporting the hypothesis that motor cortex is relatively inactive prior to S2 has not been published previously, a description of the methodology and results will be presented.

### Methods

Five monkeys *(Macaca mulatta)* were trained to press a lever during a 2,500-Hz tone to receive a 45-mg sucrose pellet. A warning stimulus (click) preceded the tone by 1 sec. A lever press between the click and the tone caused the trial to end immediately, with neither tone nor reward. The animals were trained in a heavy restraining chair to which were attached a head holder and a track designed for use with a Kopf electrode carrier. Four connectors attached to the head holder were secured to four bolts implanted in the skull of the animal, as described by RETTIG [1971]. When the subjects reached 85% correct responses, they were prepared by epidural implantation of a 1.25-cm ID stainless-steel cannula and four 8-32 stainless-steel bolts. The cannula was placed over the area of intended penetrations and closed with a Delrin cap. The bolts, with heads ground flat, were spaced around the calvarium to fit the head holder. Surface versus subcortical reference electrodes were implanted contralateral to the cannula. These, and the electrodes described below, were made of platinized [SCHWAN, 1963] platinum (90%), iridium (10%), 0.016-inch diameter wires, insulated with Epoxylite. After recovering from surgery, the animals were placed in the chair, and their heads were fixed in the holding device. An electrode consisting of four wires, with bared spots at 0–1 (No. 1), 2–3 (No. 2), 4–5 (No. 3), and 6–7 (No. 4) mm from the tip, was fixed in a Kopf electrode carrier and lowered in 1-mm increments through the cortex. A paraffin plug was used in the cannula to reduce brain pulsations. At each level, 16 or more trials were recorded for averaging. Brain electrical activity was amplified by a Brush, 8-channel, RC-coupled (time constant 1.6 sec) amplifier and stored on magnetic tape with a PI-400, 12-channel, FM recorder. Recordings were made as anterior as the frontal pole and as posterior as the precentral Rolandic gyrus.

After three penetrations through the cortex, the animal was anesthetized and perfused with saline and then formalin. The brain was removed, inspected grossly, and prepared for histological confirmation of the type of tissue penetrated and the depth reached by the electrode.

### Results

Lever press-associated events were extracted by averaging both forward and backward from correct lever presses. Activity was averaged only from those runs that showed, on stimulus-locked averages, very significant activity after S2. Figure 1 is constructed from the superimposition of the average activity from one electrode pair on the probe (No. 1 referred to No. 2, solid line) and the average of short, square-wave code pulses given at the time of correct responses (dotted line). There is an obvious similarity between the electrophysiological data and the electromechanical data, with a 160-msec lag of the electromechanical data.

In the motor cortex on the runs showing little or no CNV, such surface-positive potentials as those illustrated in figure 2 were seen commonly in well-trained monkeys. The first trace on the left, an average of 16 trials with both electrodes (No. 2 referred to No. 1) still in the epidural CSF, shows no significant activity. The second trace corresponds to the average with the tip 1 mm into the cortex. Each subsequent trace respresents the average of 8–16 trials at 1-mm decrements trough the cortex. The numbers correspond to the number of millimeters above (+) or below (—) where the surface electrode No. 2 is calculated to be. The traces to the right correspond to the averages from a single set of trials with the tip in the white matter and electrodes No. 4, No. 3, and No. 2 located +2, 0, and –2 mm above the surface. This figure demonstrates the surface-positive potential becoming a surface-negative potential (relative to the subjacent white matter) as the electrode position varies from the cerebrospinal fluid to the deep gray matter.

When the tip was referred to a distant area of white matter, the negative potential persisted to the end of the run. However, the maximum negativity clearly is nearer the more superficial electrodes than the tip, since the more superficial electrodes reflect a negativity with respect to the deeper electrode. It is possible that the reference electrodes were, in fact, recording positive shifts when the probe was at the deeper levels, that the white matter was generating a SP variation, or that there was a spread of the negative field into the subjacent white matter. The last seems the most likely explanation, since it does not require the assumption that the white matter possesses SP generators or that reference electrodes were near strong positive sources.

In the runs through motor cortex showing substantial CNVs, the termination of the CNV and the onset of the positive wave were intermingled with the slow components of the evoked response to S2, so that the potential just described was indistinguishable from other concurrent activity. Various aspects of the activity after the lever press, however, were easily distinguishable. There was a complex of surface-positive-negative-positive waves, terminating 200 msec after the lever press. In figure 3,

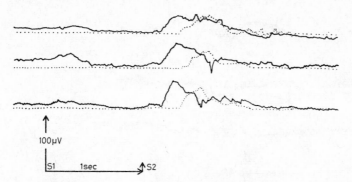

*Fig. 1.* Solid line is from electrode No. 2 referred to No. 1. Dotted line is from the output of a code channel, monitoring correct lever presses. Each pair of curves comes from the average of 16 trials at one of three progressively deeper levels. Stimuli were used to align data for averaging. In each case, electrode No. 1 is in the gray matter and electrode No. 2 is in the epicortical CSF. There is an obvious similarity in the rise time of the ECG data and the electromechanogram data. Negativity of electrode No. 1 is up.

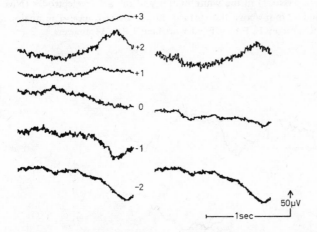

*Fig. 2.* Traces to the left are averages from one pair of electrodes (No. 2 referred to No. 1), starting above the surface of the cortex and continuing into the cortex and subjacent white matter. The numbers between the traces correspond to the number of millimeters above the surface of the cortex the active electrode is placed. The traces to the right are averages from three different pairs of electrodes (Nos. 4–1, 3–1, and 2–1) on one set of trials, with the deepest electrode (No. 1) in the white matter and the other electrodes positioned according to the numbers between the traces.

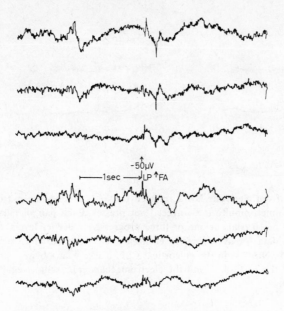

*Fig. 3.* Upper three traces: Run 5, monkey E, each an average of 16 trials with the reference electrode (No. 1) in the white matter and the active electrodes (Nos. 4, 3, and 2) +2, 0, and –2 mm above the surface. Lower three traces: The analogous averages from run 6, monkey E. FA = Feeder artifact; LP = lever press.

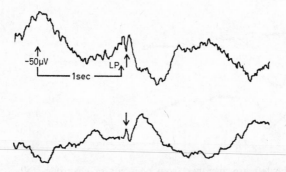

*Fig. 4.* Averages of a set of trials. Upper trace is the activity between electrodes No. 3 and No. 1. Electrode No. 3 is in the wall of sulcus arcuatus; electrode No. 1 is in the white matter below the base of sulcus arcuatus. The lower trace is the activity between electrodes No. 2 and No. 1. Electrode No. 2 is in the gray matter at the base of sulcus arcuatus. Positivity at electrode No. 1 is up. LP = Lever press artifact. Arrow indicates fast potential presumed to be evoked by the 'click' of the microswitch closure.

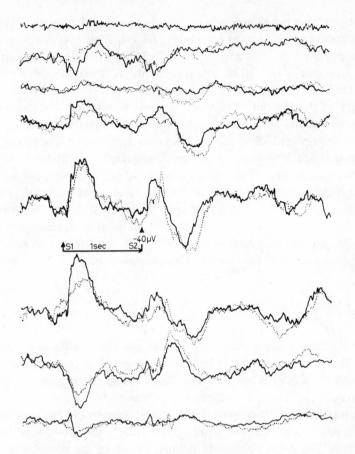

*Fig. 5.* Solid line: Averages of activity synchronized with the stimuli. Dotted line: Averages of activity synchronized with the lever press. Traces are averages of trials of run 2, monkey E. Electrode No. 3 is referred to electrode No. 1. The first trace is activity before penetration of the cortex by electrode No. 1. In the last trace, electrode No. 1 is in the white matter below the base of sulcus arcuatus and electrode No. 3 is in the deep gray of the base of the sulcus.

each trace represents one set of trials with electrode No. 4 at 2 mm, electrode No. 3 at 0 mm, and electrode No. 2 at –2 mm with respect to the surface, each referred to the tip in the subjacent white. The complex does not deteriorate or invert in run 5 (first three traces), but does show some degradation in the cortex in run 6. Also seen in these traces are some late SPs (surface-positive-negative), which invert in the outer 1 mm of cortex.

Activity in the pre-motor cortex, clearly associated with the lever press, was confined to the post-lever press period. Figure 4 illustrates a small, fast potential (arrow) and a large SP. In the first trace, electrode No. 3 (in gray matter of wall of sulcus arcuatus) is referred to electrode No. 1 (in subjacent white matter). In the second trace, electrode No. 2 (in gray matter at the bottom of sulcus arcuatus) is referred to electrode No. 1. Figure 5 shows how one can superimpose the stimulus-locked (solid line) and lever press-locked (dotted line) data and achieve a fairly good fit at the ends, with differences in the time course and amplitudes of various components. Inversions of the large, slow, lever press potential were seen to be locked to the inversion of the fast lever press potential. The fast potential bears a remarkable similarity to the click-evoked potential in time course, polarity, and levels of inversion in monkey E, penetrations 1 through 3. This potential may be an auditory EP, since there was an audible click associated with the closure of the microswitch.

## Comments

These findings indicate that there are SPs associated with motor activity and that this activity, preceding the lever press, is generally intermingled with the CNV. When recording from the motor region of well-trained monkeys, however, a surface-positive wave with a terminal negative swing was noted, with deep cortical reversal. In terms of intracellular events, this could correlate with intracellular EPSPs followed by partial repolarization. The relatively poorly defined nature of the complex suggests that it is caused by poorly synchronized inputs (the motor response involved multiple muscle groups at various time lags). When the latency of the monkey's response was greater (on the average), the lever press potential was reduced, suggesting that when the animal responded promptly, the cellular activity was more coherent.

Available data on motor potentials often is difficult to interpret because of contaminating influences. Most human studies require the subject to observe an oscilloscope in order to monitor his response mechanogram or to watch a clock in order to time his movements. Animal data usually is complicated by stimuli commanding a response or by the need to respond within a certain interval. There are post-movement stimuli in both studies, including the mechanogram trace, stereognostic feedback, microswitch closures, and oral reinforcement. These external cues may therefore be the stimuli for the motor potential, in which case the motor potentials are actually different types of sensory evoked potentials (EPs). The most careful studies, however, have revealed a positive-negative complex preceding the onset of the EMG by a latency proportional to the distance to the limb. The complex arises over contralateral motor cortex and would seem to be well correlated with excitatory axosomatic input and the spread of the excitation to the surface. Such a discrete potential complex would not be expected in the case of the data reported here, because multiple muscle systems on both sides were involved in the lever press and anticipatory reaching for the reward. Also, time locking to the EMG was not provided. In the two overtrained monkeys, the response was usually a quite discrete lever press (their paws usually rested on the lever), so there was some time locking of motor cortex input and mechanical response, but with an approximate variability of 50–100 msec.

In the stiuations wherein the CNV was prominent, i.e. in the less well-trained monkey and the pre-motor runs, the time-locked activity preceding the lever press resembled the stimulus-locked data so well that any positive-negative complex related to the response was assimilated into the falling phase of the CNV and slow evoked components of S2. Also, the motor activity that resulted in the lever press was more variable in the less-experienced monkeys, and therefore there was no consistent response time-locked to the lever press.

The fast activity following the lever press probably corresponds to an evoked response to the click of the lever press (this complex inverts much like the S1 click-evoked potential complex). The slow surface-positive activity seen in figure 5 after S2 and after the lever press appears to be of greater amplitude when averaged with respect to the lever press. A potential with similar properties was observed on the other run through Broca's area 8 into the depths of sulcus arcuatus. The polarity reversals of this slow wave correspond to those of the fast EPs, but not to the reversals of the slow EPs. The generators of this potential may be time-locked to purely internal events, partially to S2 and partially to a lever press-related event, or totally to a lever press event. The persistence of the potential in the stimulus-locked average may only reflect the rough, jittered locking of the lever press to the stimuli (see the broadened, lower-amplitude, evoked responses which result when the averages are synchronized to the lever press). The potential could well be, at least in part, the motor potential related to moving the eyes to view the feeder where the pellet should drop 0.25 sec after the lever press. It also might signify the arrival of important information – that the pellet did arrive after the lever press. The depth-negative character of this potential suggests an EPSP generator. Since the runs passed obliquely through the cortex, it cannot be said for sure what the states of the superficial layers of the cortex were, but the most intense negativity appeared to be in the middle or deep layers of gray at the bottom of the sulcus.

*Conclusions*

The overall picture of the genesis and evolution of the CNV, as illustrated in figure 6, shows a stylized slow-potential course (solid line) arising over pre-motor and motor cortex (negative up). In pre-motor areas there is a CNV early and late in learning, but in motor areas the CNV is present only initially. Stylized cortical cells illustrate the extracellular potentials measured with inhibition and excitation present during the CNV and somatic excitation at R. The appearance and disappearance of these SPs over the cortical surface probably reflect selective 'priming' of particular regions of the cerebral hemispheres, a process which is thought to be under the control of thalamic 'gating' centers and represents the acquisition of learned sensory-motor associations.

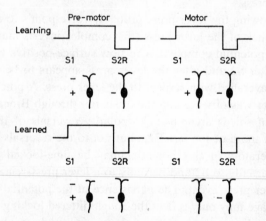

*Fig. 6.* Stylized drawing of EEG (solid line) and cellular (sketches) activity elicited by the CNV paradigm in pre-motor (left) and motor (right) cortex, early (upper) and late (lower) in conditioning. + and – refer to extracellular potentials. + is presumed to correspond with net repolarization or hyperpolarization; – is presumed to correlate with depolarization.

*References*

BORDA, R. P.: The effect of altered drive states on the contingent negative variation (CNV) in Rhesus monkeys. Electroenceph. clin. Neurophysiol. *29:* 173–180 (1970).

CREUTZFELDT, O. D.; WATANABE, S., and LUX, H. D.: Relations between EEG phenomena and potentials of single cortical cells. I. Evoked responses after thalamic and epicortical stimulation. Electroenceph. clin. Neurophysiol. *20:* 1–18 (1966).

FROST, J. D., jr. and LOW, M. D.: An electronic method for determining time-locked changes in neuronal firing rate. Electroenceph. clin. Neurophysiol. *23:* 176–178 (1967).

HABLITZ, J. J.: Operant conditioning and slow potential changes from monkey cortex. Electroenceph. clin. Neurophysiol. *34:* 399–408 (1973).

MCSHERRY, J. W.: Physiological origins of the CNV. A review. Electroenceph. clin. Neurophysiol. Suppl. *33:* 53–61 (1973).

MCSHERRY, J. W. and BORDA, R. P.: The intracortical distribution of the CNV in rhesus monkey. Electroenceph. clin. Neurophysiol. Suppl. *33:* 69–74 (1973).

REBERT, C. S.: Cortical and subcortical slow potentials in the monkey's brain during a preparatory interval. Electroenceph. clin. Neurophysiol. *33:* 389–402 (1972).

RETTIG, G. M.: A head-holding device for repeated micro-electrode studies in monkeys during operant responding. Electroenceph. clin. Neurophysiol. *30:* 462–464 (1971).

SCHWAN, H. P.: Determination of biological impedances; in NASTUK Physical techniques in biological research, vol. 6, pp. 340–343 (Academic Press, New York 1963).

STAMM, J. S. and ROSEN, S. C.: Electrical stimulation and steady potential shifts in prefrontal cortex during delayed response performance by monkeys. Acta Biol. exp., Vars. *29:* 385–399 (1969).

WALTER, W. G.: The contingent negative variation. An electro-cortical sign of sensori-motor reflex association in man. Prog. Brain Res. *22:* 364–377 (1968).

Dr. ROBERT P. BORDA, Neurophysiology Department, The Methodist Hospital, 6516 Bertner Avenue, *Houston, TX 77030* (USA). Tel. (713) 526 3311.

Dr. JOSEPH W. MCSHERRY, Department of Neurology, University of Vermont College of Medicine, *Burlington, VT 05401* (USA).

Attention, Voluntary Contraction and Event-Related Cerebral Potentials.
Prog. clin. Neurophysiol., vol. 1, Ed. J. E. DESMEDT, pp. 242–253 (Karger, Basel 1977)

# Intracerebral Slow Potential Changes in Monkeys during the Foreperiod of Reaction Time[1]

C. S. REBERT

Stanford Research Institute, Menlo Park, Calif.

Discovery of the contingent negative variation (CNV) [WALTER et al., 1964] and other event-related potentials during the last decade provided great hope that, at last, the long quest for bodily responses that mirrored particular psychological states had resulted in a significant degree of success. It became readily apparent, however, that the presence or absence of any given potential is not adequate to the prescription of any very specific molar psychological state. It is probably the case, in fact, that every subtle nuance of psychological state is associated with a unique and dynamic constellation of intracerbral relationships. Whether our technology will ever be capable of capturing the fleeting constellations associated with particular states is moot, but that appears to be the ultimate necessity in the general endeavor of correlating mind and brain. Thus, it is important to delineate as well as possible areas of the brain that are reactive in particular tasks and to assess functional intracerebral relationships. Slow potential (SP) changes have been used to pursue those goals [HAIDER et al., 1968; McCALLUM et al., 1973; IRWIN and REBERT, 1970; REBERT and IRWIN, 1969; REBERT, 1972], because SP changes are ubiquitous events in the brain that relate systematically to many physiological processes and they are often a clearer index of localized activity in the brain than the spontaneous EEG or slow-wave evoked potentials (EPs) recorded with capacity-coupled amplifiers [REBERT, 1973a].

The validity of using the SP measure as an indicator of a general change in the excitatory state of a nucleus depends on: (1) whether SPs reflect directly or indirectly neuronal activity in contrast to 'artifactual'

[1] This work was supported in part by USPHS Grant NS-08248.

events, like eye-movements, blood flow, overt movements, etc.; (2) Whether SPs recorded within a nucleus are locally generated as opposed to volume-conducted from remote generators; (3) wheter, if the SPs are locally generated, they are representative of the activity of a whole nucleus, or only a very restricted local region within a nucleus; (4) whether similar SPs in different nuclei represent similar functional conditions, or if different neuronal organizations result in a different significance of SPs among nuclei.

Studies of SP and multiple unit (MU) responses in cats and monkeys, as summarized below, indicate generally that the involvement of particular nuclei in a task, and interrelationship among nuclei can be derived from SP recording.

## Methods and Results

Procedural details of subcortical SP recordings in monkeys have been described elsewhere [REBERT, 1972] and will not be specified completely here. In general, stumptailed macaque monkeys *(Macaca arctoides)* are trained to a state of preparatory set in a cued RT task. They are taught, first, to press a bar to receive liquid reinforcement, and that response is then made contingent on the presence of a visual cue – a square aperture of light – that comes to act as an imperative stimulus (IS). Two different tones are then introduced into the situation, one of which precedes the IS by 2 sec and comes to have the properties of a warning stimulus (WS). The other, unpaired tone or discriminative stimulus (DS), provides a control for generalized effects, and introduces a discrimination into the paradigm. Anticipatory skeletal responses abort the trial. A schematic representation of the paradigm is shown in figure 1.

Data collected to date seem sufficiently reliable to allow the specification of some generalizations and tentative hypotheses. The format of this paper will be to state the generalizations and support them with illustrative material.

1) Particular loci in the brain exhibit fairly uniquely configured SP changes during the RT foreperiod, but there is great consistency in the form of such respones from one animal to another. Figure 2 shows averaged SPs from several regions in nine animals. Responses evoked from frontal cortical regions represent both motor and premotor cortices, and some differences in profile and amplitude are probably attributable to

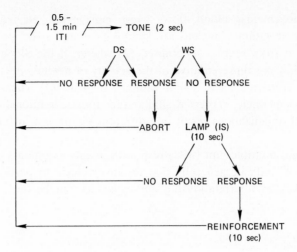

*Fig. 1.* Logic schematic indicating procedures used to establish a reaction time foreperiod paradigm for monkeys.

placement differences. The small number of responses (15) included in the averages also contributes to quantitative differences among the responses. However, in every case there is a qualitative identity of the cortical responses, the transient EP being composed of a positive-negative-positive sequence followed by a negative SP (CNV). The consistency of these cortical responses observed among a given monkey species trained under similar conditions, is less striking, however, than a nearly equal identity of such responses reported from different laboratories. Illustrations from studies by Low *et al.* [1966], Borda [1970], McSherry [1971], Hablitz [1973], Donchin *et al.* [1971], and Rebert [1972] provide evidence of a very clear and consistent sequence of potential changes in the macaque's frontal mantle during the foreperiod of RT.

SPs evoked in subcortical regions also appear to be consistent from animal to animal. Figure 2 also illustrates responses in several nonspecific reticular nuclei, and the caudate nucleus. Of considerable interest is the great similarity of responses from several nuclei that, on independent grounds, can be considered as elements of a general cerebral system, i.e. an ascending reticular activating system (ARAS). The reticular system responds quite differently than the cortex, exhibiting a simple, small, and brief positive transient followed by a rapidly developed negative SP.

The caudate nucleus shows greater variability of early transients among animals than does the cortex or nonspecific regions, but all eight

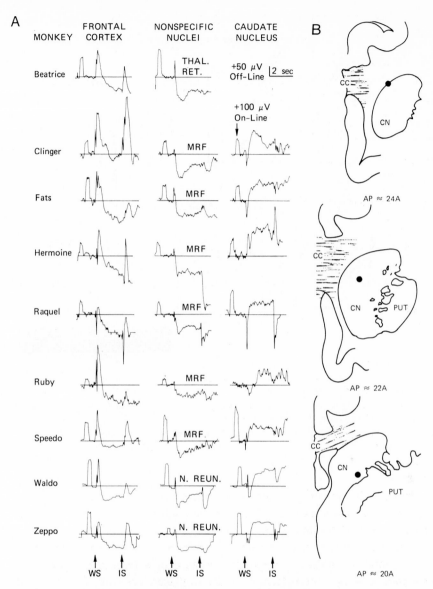

*Fig. 2. A* Averaged evoked SPs from the frontal cortex, caudate nucleus and several nonspecific nuclei, showing regional differences in polarity and waveform, but great interanimal consistency of SPs. *B* Electrode placements in different regions of the head of the caudate nucleus from which similar evoked SPs were obtained, suggesting that the nucleus in general responds in a homogeneous way. From above downwards, monkeys Raquel, Hermoine, and Waldo.

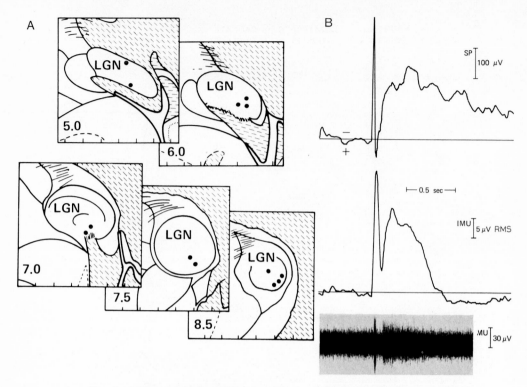

*Fig. 3. A* Electrode placements in different regions of the lateral geniculate nucleus of cats from which similar SP responses were obtained. *B* SPs, MUs, and integrated MU responses by a light flash in the cat's lateral geniculate nucleus demonstrating the association of negative SP with increased neural activity.

animals with caudate placements exhibited positive SP responses, with a fairly characteristic negative inflection and subsequent leveling of the response shortly after onset.

Demonstration of consistency of responses from a given nucleus from one animal to another is important because of a pernicious problem in stereotaxic work – the sometime failure to place electrodes similarly in all animals, resulting in unique placements in one or more animals. Evidence that responses are generally consistent from one animal to another allows the use and interpretation of results obtained in a single animal.

2) There appears to be little intranuclear differentiation in forms of the SP recorded from a given nucleus, and perhaps from general systems.

Figure 2B shows intracaudate placements that represent anterior, posterior, dorsal and ventral regions of the head of the caudate. Figure 3A shows several placements in the cat's lateral geniculate nucleus that exhibited very similar negative SP resonses to flashes of light [REBERT 1973b]. Similarly, the six MRF records shown in figure 2 were recorded from electrodes differing in their locations within the MRF.

3) SPs reflect changes in the activity of neuronal populations. Negative SPs appear to reflect increased neuronal discharge and positive SPs, decreased discharge, at least in some nuclei. Simultaneous measurements of SP and MU responses were made in the cat's lateral geniculate nucleus to test these propositions [REBERT, 1973a, b]. Figure 3B shows MU, integrated MU (IMU) and SP responses recorded from a single glass electrode [REBERT and IRWIN, 1973] in the lateral geniculate nucleus. A negative SP accompanied the increased neuronal activity produced by a light flash, whereas a positive SP accompanied decreased cellular activity produced by the presentation of steady light (fig. 4). The association of negative SPs with increased discharge was invariant. Positive SPs generally occurred in association with clear depressions of discharges, but the relationship was not as robust as that between negative SPs and increased discharge.

A modest attempt was made in one monkey to find similar effects in other nuclei during the cued RT task. The electrodes employed lacked fine tips so were not entirely appropriate for the undertaking. Negative SPs were being exhibited in the reticular formation of the animal, and positive SPs in the caudate nucleus. Results showed a fairly clear increment in activity associated with the negative MRF SP, and a very slight decline of activity in the caudate. Additional work along these lines is required to establish more definitively the SP-MU relationship, but the results from the cat's geniculate, and the suggestive effects from the monkey's MRF and caudate support the generalization that subcortically generated negative SPs in some nuclei represent an increment in neuronal activity and vice versa.

Whereas SPs appear to relate systematically to neuronal activity, the results do not suggest a direct causal relationship between the two measures. As is clear from figure 3, the profiles of the SP and IMU responses can be somewhat different. The most consistent, and nearly universal, difference in the two profiles occurs at response offset. The units typically cease firing rapidly and often show relative suppression, wherease the SP response is prolonged. Such results are compatible with the notion that

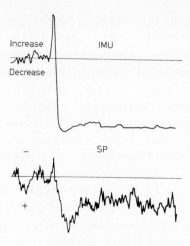

*Fig. 4.* SP and integrated MU responses from the cat's lateral geniculate nucleus demonstrating the association of positive SP with decreased neural activity produced by steady light.

the SP might reflect some combination of field potentials generated directly by neurons, and indirect consequences of neuronal effects on glial cells, mediated by a $K^+$ link [SOMJEN, 1973].

Whether any behaviorally or psychologically meaningful information is obtained from the SP response in addition to that provided by the neuronal population response is moot. If the SP does reflect glial responses, and glial potentials are some simple direct function of neuronal activity, it is not likely that much additional information is provided. However, it seems theoretically possible that glial responses could have some non-linear relationship to neuronal discharge, and might also create potential fields sufficient to feed back into the neuronal system to influence it. It would be interesting to observe whether the manipulation of experimental variables could modify SP and MU responses independently.

4) At least two major systems of the brain – the nonspecific 'arousal' system, and a rhinencephalic-related system – appear to be reciprocally responsive in the cued RT task, the former being activated during the foreperiod and the latter suppressed.

Specific structures included under the rhinencephalic rubric vary according to different authors, but include as major structures the cingulate gyrus, hippocampus, amygdala, mammillary bodies, anterior thalamus, and septum. This general system has important connections to preoptic, ventromedial and lateral hypothalamic regions, hippocampal gyrus and inferotemporal cortex, dorsal medial nucleus of the thalamus, the putamen and caudate nucleus.

Positive SPs were recorded in the foreperiod from the caudate nucleus, amygdala, preoptic area, dorsomedial nucleus, and cingulate gyrus. In contrast, negative SPs were recorded from several regions of the midbrain reticular formation, and other regions (fig. 2) comprising elements of the ARAS. This distribution of positive and negative responses during the cued RT task suggested that the two major systems delineated above were differentially reactive in the task, and reciprocally related. ROUTTENBERG [1968] has developed the general notion that the two major systems act in a reciprocal manner and he has referred to the conception as a 'two-arousal hypothesis'. The data presented here are certainly compatible with such a notion, but it is clearly a rather gross oversimplification to suggest that cerebral organization is dichotomized into general systems defined by positive or negative SPs. Also, the assignment of particular nuclei to one anatomic system or another is often ambiguous.

More precise specification of functional systems might be possible by taking into consideration parameters of the SPs other than polarity, such as form, through multivariate techniques. It is very likely that multiple systems would be delineated, and that the general excitatory level of a nucleus (polarity) would not necessarily be the most defining parameter. Some closely related nuclei can already be hypothesized to show opposite polarities in the foreperiod. For example, the caudate, which shows positive SPs, is strongly innervated by a presumed inhibitory dopaminergic input from the substantia nigra (SN) [ANDEN et al., 1964]. If the caudate-positive SP represents a response to SN inhibitory efferents, a negative SP (and increased MU activity) might be recorded from the SN.

5) Although a general interplay of broadly defined intracerebral systems appears to occur in the RT foreperiod, relationships among individual elements of the systems appear to be extremely labile. Dissociations among various brain regions in this context were first suggested by the fact that elements of the ARAS developed SP responses related to associative and discriminative factors in the task more rapidly than did the cerebral cortex (fig. 5A). In another group of animals, the MRF also showed a clear discrimination between the WS and DS during mid-training whereas the cortex did not (fig. 5B). Correlations among placements of SP amplitude across trials indicated that the caudate and amygdala varied together whereas the MRF and cortex were independent.

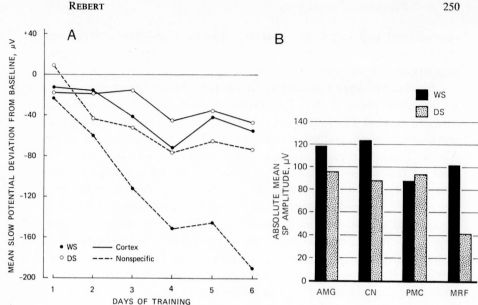

*Fig. 5. A* Mean amplitude changes over the course of the first six training days of SP responses recorded from the frontal cortex and nonspecific projection nuclei demonstrating a dissociation of cortical and nonspecific SP responses. *B* Differential SP responses to warning and discriminative stimuli in the amygdala (AMG) caudate nucleus (CN) premotor cortex (PMC), and midbrain reticular formation (MRF). The MRF shows a large difference in SP amplitude to the two stimuli whereas the cortex shows none.

## Discussion

The following data suggests that SP measures are significant local events unrelated to volume-conducted remote potentials: (1) SPs were evoked from only some placements in a given animal; (2) a variety of waveforms were observed within individual animals; (3) both positive and negative potentials were recorded at different sites in individual monkeys, and from proximate placements in some regions of the cat's brain [RE-BERT and IRWIN, 1969]; (4) development of SPs from various nuclei occurred at different rates during training; (5) slight variations in placement of electrodes aimed at the same site in different animals resulted in different responses when the electrode was placed in a different structure, whereas similar responses were recorded from electrodes placed in homologous structures; (6) an active reference was easily detected in one animal in which the reference was in the cingulate gyrus; (7) both the initial EP complex and the subsequent SP changes recorded referentially in this study from the cortex are identical in form to those recorded transcortically by DONCHIN et al. [1971] in their equivalent task F; (8) eye movements that occurred during a trial were rapid, variable and uncorrelated with SPs; (9) SPs appear to be closely related directly or indirectly to neuronal population discharges; (10) flash-evoked SP and MU in the cat's lateral geniculate nucleus were not observed until the electrode was within about 0.5 mm of the nucleus; (11) SP and MU responses may reflect better than either slow wave EEG or EP the distribution of cortical activity associated with tonic sensory stimulation [GUMMIT, 1961; STARR and LIVINGSTON, 1963]; and (12) subcortically recorded SPs relate meaningfully to anatomical organization under acute conditions of simultaneous stimulation and recording [HAYWARD et al., 1966]. Thus, an evoked SP indicates that a significant functional change occurred in a nucleus. The magnitude of the SP reponse is also related to the degree of functional alteration. The sizes of SP and MU responses in the cat's lateral geniculate nucleus to light flashes, for example, are both a function of background illumination [ARDUINI and PINNEO, 1963; REBERT, 1973a].

In these studies, the SP measure, like the CNV, changes systematically as the animals have increased experience in the task and during extinction. The labile internuclear relationships reflected by the SP responses thus appear to be valid. In contrast to physiological studies that indicate a very close interlocking of cortex and MRF [cf. ARDUINI, 1958], the analysis of responses obtained in the psycho-physiological paradigm reported here reveals a nearly complete dissociation of the MRF and frontal cortex. The results call into question inferences made from human CNV studies about reticular mechanisms involved in CNV genesis [MCADAM, 1969], and call for more realistic and differentiated model of the neural mechanisms regulating the cerebral electrogenesis [cf. SKINNER and YINGLING, this volume].

Some of the intracerebral patterns of SP distribution indicated here for the monkey have been found to be essentially the same in humans. MCCALLUM et al. [1973] reported that positive potentials occurred in or near the human caudate nucleus, whereas negative SPs were observed in the reticular formation. The form of the SPs were also similar, the caudate exhibiting rather slowly developing responses and the MRF short-latency, fast rising ones. HAIDER et al. [1968] have also reported that several human thalamic nuclei exhibit SP responses during the RT foreperiod, and have suggested that the cortical CNV is closely linked to activity in the ventral thalamus. The concordance between available results from the human and monkey in terms of SP distribution, polarity, latency, and general waveform is important in indicating the relevance of monkey-CNV studies to human CNV work.

With respect to the validity of using SP responses to index localized cerebral activity, the data presented above indicate that the SPs recorded in the cued RT task reflect neuronal excitability and are locally generated within a nucleus yet reflect the overall activity of at least some nuclei. In general, the studies of subcortical SP changes in the cued RT task indicate which regions of the brain are responsive in the situation, and which covary or are relatively independent. Of course, it is clear that whereas macro-responses like SPs or multiple units may indicate that a given nucleus is more or less active during some period of time, and may reveal gross system interactions, such responses do not reflect the more subtle patterning of neuronal interaction within a nucleus. However, the situation is analogous to machine indicators that reflect the participation of various computer elements at any time, yet do not indicate the details of the program that is running, and it seems quite possible that one could eventually infer from the patterns of gross indicators studied that one or another program was running, and predictions about machine outputs could be made. Despite some difficulties, therefore, it is meaningful to attempt to define, in terms of regional activity, general cerebral systems that operate in particular behavioral situations.

## References

ANDEN, N. E.; CARLSSON, A.; DAHLSTROM, A.; FUXE, K.; HILLARP, N. A., and LARSSON, K.: Demonstration and mapping out of the nigro-neostriatal dopamine neurons. Life Sci. *3:* 523–530 (1964).

ARDUINI, A.: Enduring potential changes evoked in the cerebral cortex by stimulation of brain stem reticular formation and thalamus; in JASPER, PROCTOR, KNIGHTON, NOSHAY and COSTELLO Reticular formation of the brain, pp. 333–350 (Little, Brown, Boston 1958).

ARDUINI, A. and PINNEO, L. R.: The tonic activity of the lateral geniculate nucleus in dark and light adaptation. Arch. ital. Biol. *101:* 493–507 (1963).

BORDA, R. P.: Drive and performance related aspects of the CNV in rhesus monkeys. Electroenceph. clin. Neurophysiol. *20:* 173–180 (1970).

DONCHIN, E.; OTTO, D.; GERBRANDT, L. K., and PRIBRAM, K. H.: While a monkey waits. Electrocortical events recorded during the foreperiod of a reaction time study. Electroenceph. clin. Neurophysiol. *31:* 115–127 (1971).

GUMMIT, R. J.: The distribution of direct current responses evoked by sounds in the auditory cortex of the cat. Electroenceph. clin. Neurophysiol. *13:* 889–895 (1961).

HABLITZ, J. J.: Operant conditioning and slow potential changes from monkey cortex. Electroenceph. clin. Neurophysiol. *34:* 399–408 (1973).

HAIDER, M.; GANGLBERGER, J. A., and GROLL-KNAPP, E.: Computer analyzed thalamic potentials and their relation to expectancy waves in man. Acta neurol. latinoamer *14:* 132–137 (1968).

HAYWARD, J. N.; FAIRCHILD, M. D., and STUART, D. G.: Hypothalamic and cortical D-C potential changes induced by stimulation of the midbrain reticular formation. Expl Brain Res. *1:* 205–219 (1966).

IRWIN, D. A. and REBERT, C. S.: Slow potential changes in cat brain during classical appetitive conditioning of jaw movements using two levels of reward. Electroenceph. clin. Neurophysiol. *28:* 119–126 (1970).

LOW, M. D.; BORDA, R. P., and KELLAWAY, P.: 'Contingent negative variation' in rhesus monkeys: an EEG sign of a specific mental process. Percept. Motor Skills *22:* 443–446 (1966).

MCADAM, D. W.: Increases in CNS excitability during negative cortial slow potentials in man. Psychon. Sci. *26:* 216–219 (1969).

MCCALLUM, W. C.; PAPAKOSTOPOULOS, D.; GOMBI, R.; WINTER, A. L.; COOPER, R., and GRIFFITH, H. B.: Event related slow potential changes in human brain stem. Nature, Lond. *242:* 465–467 (1973).

MCSHERRY, J. W.: Intracortical origin of the contingent negative variation in the rhesus monkey; doct. diss., Houston (1971).

REBERT, C. S.: Cortical and subcortical slow potentials in the monkey's brain during a preparatory interval. Electroenceph. clin. Neurophysiol. *33:* 389–402 (1972).

REBERT, C. S.: A technique for simultaneous measurement of DC and multiple unit responses. Electroenceph. clin. Neurophysiol. *34:* 326–328 (1973a).

REBERT, C. S.: Slow potential correlates of neuronal population responses in the cat's lateral geniculate nucleus. Electroenceph. clin. Neurophysiol. *35:* 511–515 (1973b).

REBERT, C. S. and IRWIN, D. A.: Slow potential changes in cat brain during classical appetitive and aversive conditioning of jaw movement. Electroenceph. clin. Neurophysiol. *27:* 152–161 (1969).

ROUTTENBERG, A.: The two-arousal hypothesis: reticular formation and limbic system. Psychol. Rev. *75:* 51–80 (1968).

SOMJEN, G.: Electrogenesis of sustained potentials. Prog. Neurobiol., vol. 1, pp. 199–235 (1973).

STARR, A. and LIVINGSTON, R. B.: Long-lasting nervous system responses to prolonged sound stimulation in waking cats. J. Neurophysiol. *26:* 416–431 (1963).

Dr. CHARLES S. REBERT, Neurophysiology Program, Stanford Research Institute, *Menlo Park, CA 94025* (USA). Tel. (415) 326 6200.

# Subject Index

Activation pattern 53
Akinesia 146, 151
Alertness 8, 58, 79, 86
Alpha rhythm 56, 135, 142, 159
Alternation task 51
Anxiety 60
Artifacts 8, 22, 124, 133, 152
Attention 8, 30, 52, 98, 141, 182, 231, 242
Augmenting responses 35, 65, 77
Autonomic regulation 59
Averaging 22, 132, 143, 152, 233
Aversive conditioning 60, 92

Ballistic movements 143
Bandpass 5, 13, 20, 101, 192, 212
Basal ganglia 146, 151
Behaviorism 61
Bereitschaftspotential 14, 124, 133, 152, 164, 190
Blockings of amplifier 14, 24
Brainstem EPs 15, 25
Bulbar synchronizing system 33

Calibration 6
Carbon dioxide in blood 148
Cardiac arrhythmias 61
Centrifugal gating of input 85
Cerebellar input to VL thalamic nucleus 87
Cerebellum 148
Chopper-stabilized amplifier 14
CNV 4, 14, 30, 63, 91, 98, 123, 126, 136, 180, 190

Conditioning 48
Consciousness 31
Control of sensory input 54, 95
Covert motor readiness 127
Cryoprobe 32

Data presentation 8
Deafferentation of limb 219
Debriefing subjects 8
Depth recording 165, 231, 242
Differential SPs with unimanual tasks 125
Disjunctive reaction time task 109
Duality of thalamic synchronizing mechanisms 56

EEG synchronization 88
Electrodermal potentials 21, 133
Electrodes 4, 20
Electro-oculograms 5, 22, 101, 119, 133, 152, 192, 213
Electroretinogram 128
Environment of subject 4, 25
Epilepsy 166
Expectancy 30, 79, 83, 98, 215, 232
Extinction of behavioral response 54
Extracephalic references 24, 133
Eye movements 4, 22, 119, 133

Fast EP components 20
Feedback control of sensory input 53, 84
Filters 5, 13

H2